Reducing the Carcinogenic Risks in Industry

OCCUPATIONAL SAFETY AND HEALTH

A Series of Reference Books and Textbooks
on Occupational Hazards ● Safety ● Health ●
Fire Protection ● Security ● and Industrial Hygiene

Series Editor
ALAN L. KLING
Loss Prevention Consultant
Jamesburg, New Jersey

Other Volumes in Preparation

Reducing the Carcinogenic Risks in Industry

edited by

Paul F. Deisler, Jr.

Shell Oil Company
Houston, Texas

MARCEL DEKKER, INC.   New York and Basel

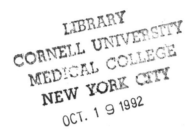
Library of Congress Cataloging in Publication Data

Main entry under title:

Reducing the carcinogenic risks in industry.

(Occupational safety and health ; 9)
Includes index.
1. Cancer—Prevention. 2. Occupational diseases—
Prevention. 3. Industrial toxicology. I. Deisler,
Paul F., Jr. -[date] . II. Series: Occupational Safety
and health (Marcel Dekker, Inc.) ; v. 9. [DNLM:
1. Carcinogens. 2. Neoplasms—prevention & control.
3. Occupational Diseases—chemically induced.
4. Occupational Diseases—prevention & control.
W1 OC597M v.9 / WA 465 R321]
RC268.R43   1984   362.1'96994   84—17448
ISBN 0—8247—7250—4

MARCEL DEKKER, INC.
270 Madison Avenue, New York, New York 10016

Current printing (last digit):
10 9 8 7 6 5 4 3 2 1

PRINTED IN THE UNITED STATES OF AMERICA

FOREWORD

I feel honored by the invitation to write a foreword for this praiseworthy effort by Dr. Paul Deisler and his coauthors. I am convinced *Reducing the Carcinogenic Risks in Industry* will make a substantial contribution to the amelioration of the situation with which it is concerned.

This book leaves one with an overall impression of abundant good sense and reasonableness that match the excellent quality of the various contributions. In comparison with some recent books on related topics, there is no less realism about the problems, no less determination to work toward effective solutions. But all this in the absence of rancor, of vitriolic attacks, and without impugning the integrity and the motives of all save the true believers—a refreshing and welcome change!

So much for the tone of the book. Now for the substance. The treatment of the subject follows a logical progression, from outlining the existing potential cancer risks to considering the strategy for diminishing the incidence of industrial cancer. The means for achieving this end are each analyzed in turn: toxicology and epidemiology, the federal research effort in this direction, and the part played by the practitioners of industrial hygiene. At this point the reader is apt to wonder: Yes, it all sounds very well, but does it work? A number of examples are cited that point to ways in which cancer risk in the workplace has been controlled and reduced, often by voluntary action on the part of enlightened industry, at other times as a consequence of effective intervention by the Occupational Safety and Health Administration. The situation with regard to cancer risk in Western European industry is presented for purposes of comparison. The final chapter in this comprehensive treatise deals with the developing partnership of science, policy, and the law. There is a note of optimism that such cooperation will take the place of confrontation and ultimately help to reduce the risk of cancer in the workplace. Echoing the theme of Milton Wessel's works, this chapter offers the hope that good science will prevail: "In both law and science, the more that is known about the mechanism of the disease or injury, the greater the assurance of correctness of the decision."

Mention of the importance of understanding the mechanism of toxic action brings to mind two scientific organizations to which reference is made in this book, and with which I have had the good fortune to have been associated in earlier days. The British Industrial Biological Research Association (BIBRA) is an endeavor jointly supported by government and industry. It enjoys worldwide respect. The Chemical Industry Institute of Toxicology (CIIT) is financed entirely by United States industry, and is equally committed to the goals of objectivity and scientific excellence. Both have contributed substantially to the reduction of cancer risk in the workplace, the home, and the environment by developing toxicological data and then performing that most difficult of tasks: doggedly pursuing an understanding of the underlying mechanisms that are responsible for the observed effects. Few research laboratories have comparable standards of excellence, consistent support, and the scale of multidisciplinary staff and facilities to make such contributions to the reduction of cancer risk.

My colleagues and I in the fields of community and occupational medicine have reason to be grateful for the comprehensive coverage of the subject of carcinogenic risks in industry and the means employed to reduce these hazards. Our students, residents, and fellows will be greatly helped by the broad perspective and sage advice that is offered. The real audience for this book, however, extends beyond academia, or the medical establishment, to the public at large. They will be the ultimate beneficiaries.

Leon Golberg
Professor of Community
and Occupational Medicine
Duke University Medical Center
Durham, North Carolina

PREFACE

The discovery that cancer can be caused by prolonged contact with soot was made 200 years ago. It is only in the last decade or so, however, that the possibilities for other man-made agents to cause cancer have penetrated the public consciousness.

The reaction to this occurrence has been powerful and widespread. It has accelerated scientific developments, given impetus to the passage of far-reaching legislation, and led to the development of regulations, regulatory policies, and private initiatives aimed at reducing or eliminating cancer in, or associated with, industry. Governmental, academic, and industrial organizations have all entered the field and the variety of approaches, in the United States and elsewhere, is very great.

It is not possible, in a single short volume, to cover all aspects of this broad activity. The 11 chapters in this volume, each written by contributors who are actively involved in various aspects of the problem of industrially derived cancer risk, cannot represent the full spectrum of approaches, philosophies, controversies, or contributions in this field. They do cover many important areas, in the United States and Western Europe, ranging from defining the nature and scope of the current problem through the status of philosophical, scientific, and technical developments and their application by government and industry, to the developing partnership between science, policy, and the law. Readers of this volume who are expert in one or another of the areas represented will, I hope, appreciate the chapters dealing with their areas and gain additional insights as they read the other chapters. The work is not intended solely for such experts, however, but also for teachers, scientists, technologists, governmental officials, managers, and other informed and interested individuals.

It is clear that these 11 chapters are but a sampling of the total activity; the picture they paint is of a major societal problem in the process of being solved. It is not a picture of unity of action or viewpoint, however, for there is much uncertainty; consequently, the solutions are varied and estimates of the probabilities of success—and what constitutes success—are equally diverse. Indeed, while all the contributors agree that there are true risks to be dealt with, there is no similar agreement on how to go about it, or how far one can or should go in reducing the risk from a particular hazard. It is hoped that the reader will emerge not only with an understanding of the complexities involved, but also with some sense of progress and, even though the story is far from complete, with the feeling that continued effort will bring down the overall risk of cancer from industrial sources to the point that it no longer need be either the cause celebre or the cause of fear that it is today.

It has been a pleasure to help put this work together; in so doing I have had the invaluable assistance of Miss Eula McMurry in ensuring that what my eye missed, hers caught, and in handling a remarkable flow of paper in an orderly way. That assistance is gratefully acknowledged.

Paul F. Deisler, Jr.

CONTRIBUTORS

Robert C. Barnard, B.Cl., M.A. Senior Partner, Cleary, Gottlieb, Steen, and Hamilton, Washington, D.C. and General Counsel, American Industrial Health Council, Washington, D.C.

Jacqueline K. Corn, D.A. Assistant Professor, Environmental Health Sciences, The Johns Hopkins University School of Hygiene and Public Health, Baltimore, Maryland

Morton Corn, Ph.D., M.S., B.Ch.E.* Professor and Director, Division Environmental Health Engineering, Environmental Health Sciences, The Johns Hopkins University School of Hygiene and Public Health, Baltimore, Maryland

Paul F. Deisler, Jr., Ph.D. Vice President, Health, Safety, and Environment, Shell Oil Company, Houston, Texas

James E. Gibson, Ph.D. Vice President and Director of Research, Chemical Industry Institute of Toxicology, Research Triangle Park, North Carolina

Michael Gough, Ph.D. Senior Associate, Office of Technology Assessment, Congress of the United States, Washington, D.C.

---

*Formerly Assistant Secretary of Labor for Occupational Safety and Health, Washington, D.C.

John Higginson, M.D.* Senior Scientist, Universities Associated for Research and Education in Pathology, Inc., Bethesda, Maryland

Bruce W. Karrh, M.D. Vice President, Safety, Health, and Environmental Affairs, E.I. du Pont de Nemours and Company, Wilmington, Delaware

Howard L. Kusnetz, P.E., C.I.H.† Manager, Safety and Industrial Hygiene, Shell Oil Company, Houston, Texas

William W. Lowrance, Ph.D.‡ Senior Fellow and Director, Life Sciences and Public Policy Program, The Rockefeller University, New York, New York

Jeremiah Lynch,† Manager, Industrial Hygiene, Medicine and Environmental Affairs Department, Exxon Chemical Company, East Millstone, New Jersey

Robert A. Neal, Ph.D. President, Chemical Industry Institute of Toxicology, Research Triangle Park, North Carolina

Duurt Frederik Rijkels, M.D. Head, Health, Safety, and Environment Division, Shell Internationale Petroleum Maatschappij B.V., The Hague, The Netherlands

Leonard A. Sagan, M.D. Senior Scientist, Energy Analysis and Environment Division, Electric Power Research Institute, Palo Alto, California

Chris G. Whipple, Ph.D. Technical Manager, Energy Study Center, Electric Power Research Institute, Palo Alto, California

---

*Formerly Director, International Agency for Research on Cancer, World Health Organization, Lyon, France.
†Engineering Director, U.S. Public Health Service. (Retired.)
‡Formerly Special Assistant to U. S. Undersecretary of State for Security Assistance, Science, and Technology, and Member of the faculties of Harvard and Stanford Universities, and Resident Fellow, National Academy of Sciences.

CONTENTS

1

EXISTING RISKS FOR CANCER

John Higginson*
*Universities Associated for Research and Education in Pathology, Inc.
Bethesda, Maryland*

*Formerly Director International Agency for Research on Cancer, World Health Organization, Lyon, France

1

I. INTRODUCTION

Cancer comprises a variety of diseases to which nearly all organs of the body are susceptible. Essentially, the disease consists of a change in one of the cells within an organ whereby the cell reproduced uncontrollably. If it spreads to other parts of the body, it can eventually kill the patient. Although the fundamental molecular biochemical changes at the cellular level are not yet understood, there is enough similarity between different types of tumors to justify their inclusion under the overall term "cancer."

In the 18th and 19th centuries, with high mortality due to tuberculosis, smallpox, and other diseases, cancer was a comparatively rare disease, believed to be possibly hereditary or an inevitable accompaniment of aging. Accordingly, there was relatively little interest in the possibilities of prevention, although in 1775 Percival Pott, a London surgeon, suggested that scrotal cancer in chimney sweeps might be caused by soot and be controlled through improved hygiene [1]. In 1834 in Verona, Italy, Stern demonstrated that sexual behavior was related to the development of cancer of the breast and uterus [1]. Later, doctors came to associate cancer with modern industrial societies, believing that it was rare in primitive communities such as Africa. At the beginning of the 20th century, a number of cancers were identified as causally associated with exposure to chemicals in certain occupations, such as bladder cancer in dye workers and skin tumors due to exposure to shale oil. At the same time, modern experimental cancer research began to develop with the demonstration that chemicals could cause cancer in animals and, thus, possibly warn of human risk. Radiation and ultraviolet light were recognized as carcinogenic stimuli. In the 1950s it was confirmed that cultural habits, notably tobacco and alcohol, but also general diet and behavior, were also associated with varying cancer risks. Today it is accepted that 80–90% of cancers are causally associated to a varying degree with many different types of environmental factors [1–4]. In evaluating the effects of the environment on disease, it is necessary to identify and measure not only the suspected environmental factors concerned, but also the responses—in this case, cancer. The objective of this chapter is to outline those environmental risks believed to be responsible for the greater part of the cancer burden within a modern industrial society.

II. THE ENVIRONMENT

The effects of the environment on disease have been accepted since Hippocrates, the term "environment" implying all exogenous factors which impinge on humans. While this wide definition is accepted for most diseases, such as heart disease, there has been a recent tendency to limit the term for neoplastic diseases to synthetic chemicals. In the present discussion the term is used in its widest sense and subclassified as follows for convenience.

A. The Chemical Environment

While the effects of nearly all carcinogenic stimuli at a fundamental or molecular level can or will be describable in biochemical terms, in practice it is convenient to limit "chemical environment" to discrete exogenous chemicals or mixtures of chemicals, whether man-made or of natural origin. Humans have long been exposed to numerous cancer-producing chemicals arising from dust, fungal contaminants, dietary constituents, and burning organic matter, to name a few. The biological impact of most such compounds remains poorly understood, and their importance on background cancer rates remains to be determined. However, aflatoxin, a mycotoxin, has been shown to be related to liver cancer in Africa and Asia.

In recent years, much attention has been directed to the many chemicals that have been synthesized since the mid-19th century, of which 30,000 are in common use. Humans may be exposed to such chemicals not only in the general or ambient environment, but also in higher doses in their personal environment as a result of occupation (Table 1), medical therapy (Table 2), cultural habits, and other factors (Table 3). Most of our knowledge of the carcinogenic action of chemicals has come through examination of exposures to such high exposures [5]. Much less is known about the effects of such chemicals at low levels in the general environment, such as in water, air, and food. These effects are very difficult to discern and measure, but such low-level exposures are the focus of most public concern.

Table 1 Established Carcinogens and Carcinogenic Risk Factors in Humans

Occupational	
Agent or occupation	Site
Aromatic amines	
4-Aminodiphenyl	Bladder
Benzidine	Bladder
2-Naphthylamine	Bladder
Arsenic	Skin, lung
Asbestos	Lung, pleura, peritoneum
Benzene	Marrow
Bis(chloromethyl) ether	Lung
Cadmium	Prostate
Chromium	Lung
Furniture manufacture (hardwood)	Nasal sinuses
Ionizing radiations	Marrow and probably all other sites
Isopropyl alcohol manufacture	Nasal sinuses
Leather goods manufacture	Nasal sinuses
Mustard gas	Larynx, lung
Nickel	Nasal sinuses, lung
Polycyclic hydrocarbons	Skin, scrotum, lung
Ultraviolet light	Skin, lip
Vinyl chloride	Liver (angiosarcoma)

Table 2 Established Carcinogens and Carcinogenic Risk Factors in Humans

Medical therapy	
Agent	Site
Alkylating agents	
Cyclophosphamide	Bladder
Melphalan	Marrow
Arsenic	Skin, lung
Busulphan	Marrow
Chlornaphazine	Bladder
Immunosuppressive drugs	Reticuloendothelial system
Ionizing radiations	Marrow and probably all other sites
Estrogens	
Unopposed	Endometrium
Transplacental (DES)	Vagina
Phenacetin	Kidney (pelvis)
Polycyclic hydrocarbons	Skin, scrotum, lung
Steroids	
Anabolic (oxymetholone)	Liver
Contraceptives	Liver (hamartoma)

B. The Physical Environment

The carcinogenic effect of ionizing radiation was very early recognized among those involved in developing radiology. Today, the most important source of added exposures to the general public still comes from diagnostic medical procedures. Some added exposures also occur in the workplace. Although very low exposures to ionizing radiation in the background environment is widely recognized, no one is quite certain of their impact on human cancer, but they probably cause much less than 1% of all cancers. Solar radiation is the major cause of cancer of the skin, and exposure and resultant skin cancer have been increasing in recent years, especially among younger people, due to changing cultural habits in western countries.

Table 3 Established Carcinogens and Carcinogenic Risk Factors in Humans

Diet, behavior, and lifestyle	
Agent	Site
Aflatoxin	Liver
Alcoholic drinks	Mouth, pharynx, larynx, esophagus, liver
Chewing betel, tobacco, lime	Mouth
Overnutrition (causing obesity)	Endometrium, gallbladder
Reproductive history	
Late age at 1st pregnancy	Breast
Zero or low parity	Ovary
Parasites	
Schistosoma haematobium	Bladder
Chlonorchis sinensis	Liver (cholangioma)
Sexual promiscuity	Cervix uteri
Smoking tobacco	Mouth, pharynx, larynx, lung, esophagus, bladder
Ultraviolet light	Skin, lip
Virus (hepatitis B)	Liver (hepatoma)

C. The Biological Environment

The role of exogenous viruses in human cancer remains somewhat controversial. There is evidence, however, that viruses may be involved in certain rare leukemias: in a tumor of lymphatic tissue in children, especially in Africa; in tumors of the nasopharynx in China; and in liver cancer in Africa. It has been suggested that viral infection is also important in cancer of the uterine cervix, a very common cancer in women in Africa and Latin American, which is also significantly modified by behavioral patterns. On the other hand, there are a number of parasitic diseases associated with cancer, notably schistosomiasis, widespread in Africa, the Middle East, and Asia. Another parasite, a liver fluke, is associated with liver cancer in Southeast Asia.

Recently, the recognition that certain oncogenes occur in human tumors and some appear similar to certain cancer-inducing viruses in animals has raised the question of the role of such oncogenes in human cancer. Such genes are under intensive scrutiny as to their nature, origin, and mode of action, but it appears that, for the moment, the fundamental question will remain of how and what environmental factors trigger or activate oncogenes. Viruses have been implicated in a certain type of leukemia and possibly in Kaposi's sarcomas which are associated with acquired immune deficiency syndrome (AIDS), a syndrome in which horizontal transference has been reported.

D. The Cultural and Behavioral Environment

This environment can be divided into clearly defined cultural habits, such as cigarette smoking and alcoholic beverage intake, and less clearly defined risk factors related to diet and sexual behavior (Table 3). Both groups, but especially the latter, are often described as "lifestyle." A major step in the potential control of human disease in recent years has been the recognition that a number of cultural habits may be hazardous. Of these, the most important is cigarette smoking. In addition, excessive drinking of alcoholic beverages has been shown to be an important factor in certain cancers, such as mouth, esophagus, and liver. In India, betel chewing is responsible for cancer of the mouth and upper digestive tract.

It has also been shown that certain types of sexual behavior and reproductive factors may be risk factors in tumors of the breast, uterus, and ovaries, such as age of first pregnancy, number of children, age of onset and frequency of sexual intercourse, and so forth. The mechanisms whereby such behavior modifies cancer incidence are imperfectly understood, but may be linked to subtle biochemical changes that modify rates of hormone metabolism in the liver and other organs, affecting DNA repair, gene enhancement, and other mechanisms.

The most important elements of "lifestyle," however, probably relate to dietary habits [2–4,6]. Dietary variables include free-formed potential carcinogens such as hydrocarbons, protein pyrolyzates, or food additives; carcinogen precursors, such as secondary amines and nitrates; and such natural contaminants as aflatoxin. There is little evidence that the natural substances, apart from aflatoxin in Africa and Asia, have had a major impact on cancer patterns in most areas, especially in industrial countries.

Recent research has concentrated on the indirect effects of various nutrients and nonnutrients. Such studies cover the type and relative proportion of different foods, such as the ratio of saturated to unsaturated fats, or the presence of trace elements. Although the role of certain fats has been well established in experimental carcinogenesis, their significance in humans remains somewhat controversial. Studies relating cancers of the breast and colon to meat, fat, and calorie intake have not been supported by other studies populations of Mormons and Roman Catholic nuns. Further, the role of fecal flora is poorly understood. In conclusion, the exact role of diet has not been consistently demonstrated or defined, and thus while most authorities regard diet as of major importance for many cancers, its contribution to the human cancer burden remains uncertain.

Non-nutrient dietary factors may also affect carcinogenesis, and there is evidence that low fiber intake may significantly enhance cancer of the colon. In contrast, dietary factors may inhibit cancer development. Thus, while green vegetables contain promoters and enhancers, they also contain inactivating and inhibiting factors such as vitamin A or antioxidants. The level of caloric intake also modifies cancer patterns, most cancer rates being higher in obese individuals. Thus, diet is no longer considered solely in terms of food additives or ingested carcinogens.

Investigations from a number of sources have confirmed that tumors of endocrine-dependent organs depend on environmental factors, including behavior, the effects of which may become apparent only over several generations. These factors include early age at first pregnancy, which seems to protect against breast cancer. Although it is possible to speculate that such culturally determined factors may lead to subtle change in hormonal status, there is also a close interrelationship between diet and behavior, which makes evaluation of each component difficult to determine. Thus, diet is a significant factor in the determination of height, weight, and age of menarche, all of which have been described as risk factors for cancer of the breast and endometrium.

Lastly, there is unequivocal evidence that noncarcinogenic chemicals may interact within the body to form carcinogens such as N-nitroso compounds from dietary nitrates and secondary amines. However, the significance of such endogenous carcinogen formation in humans remains to be demonstrated, although it is widely suspected as important. It is therefore impossible to speak of the cancer risk of any dietary constituent with exactitude, recognizing that diet implies the summation of a wide range of different risks which may directly or indirectly affect the action of other carcinogens.

III. CARCINOGENS AND CARCINOGENIC RISK FACTORS

From the viewpoint of cancers of known and suspected etiology, cancer causing factors in the environment can be classified into two major groups: (1) defined carcinogenic stimuli and (2) carcinogenic risk factors.

A. Defined Carcinogenic Stimuli

The concept of a defined carcinogen (chemical or physical) is widely understood and can be examined by standard epidemiological and other techniques. It is customary to divide such stimuli into initiators such as vinyl chloride, which are believed to significantly modify the nuclear material in the cell (possibly by oncogene activation) and eventually produce irreversible changes, and those which are believed to affect the later stages of carcinogenesis by as yet unknown mechanisms and which do not necessarily damage the genetic cellular material directly. The latter are sometimes described as promoters such as certain hormones. The distinction between these two types of carcinogenic factors is not yet clear, and while differences in mechanisms may be unimportant at high exposures, they may be of significance in interpreting potential effects at low doses. For example, cigarette smoke contains both initiating and promoting factors, but the relative role of each is not clearly established. For practical or operational purposes, discrete promoting chemicals for example, hormones, can be described as "operational carcinogens," but such a term might be unsuitable to describe unsaturated fats.

B. Carcinogenic Risk Factors

There are, however, a number of identified and definable risk factors that are associated with an increased cancer risk but that cannot readily be called carcinogens. Such factors include dietary fiber deficiency, excessive dietary fat, obesity, and such behavioral patterns as age at first pregnancy. Eventually, the role of such factors may be describable in terms of chemical or metabolic mechanisms that might relate to multistage or cocarcinogenesis in humans. Such factors are believed to be important for a wide range of cancers.

C. Multifactorial Causes and Predominant or   Avoidable Cause

A carcinogenic factor may be so predominant that in its absence a measurable percentage of a particular cancer would not occur, and thus it can be regarded for practical purposes as a predominant or avoidable cause of that cancer [3,4]. This does not mean that other factors may not play a contributory role. The recognition, however, of avoidable or predominant factors allows the development of effective public health strategies. Thus, cigarettes can be regarded as the practical or avoidable cause of 80–90% of all cancers of the lung and a high percentage of cancers of the esophagus, irrespective of the mechanisms whereby they induce cancer (Table 4). Other factors such as asbestos in the case of lung cancer or ethanol in cancer of the esophagus, can multiply the effects of cigarettes and thus be regarded as avoidable causes for these sites.

In occupational or medically induced exposures, an identified factor may be controlled and eliminated. In contrast, the definition and control of those carcinogenic risk factors which affect a large part of the population may require many more years of research, since in most cases their biological impact or exact nature

Table 4 Percentage Impact of Excess Deaths
Due to Cancer in Smokers

Site	Male	Female
Lung	82.8	43.1
Esophagus	66.7	50.0
Mouth and larynx	81.3	44.4
Bladder	48.8	9.6
Pancreas	47.7	11.0
All cancers	34.5	5.4

Source: Ref. [9].

Table 5 Estimates of Proportion of Avoidable Cancers

	United States deaths [4]		Birmingham, England cases [3]	
	Best estimate both sexes	Range	Male	Female
Tobacco	30	24–40	30	7
Alcohol	3	2–40	5	3
Lifestyle				
Diet	35	10–79 ⎫	30	63
Reproductive habits	7	7–13 ⎭		
Food additives	<1	−5–2	—	—
Occupation	4	2–8	6	2
Iatrogenic	1	0.5–3	1	1
Pollution	2	<1–5	—	—
Industrial products[a]	<1	<1–2	—	—
Geophysical (incl. UV light ionizing reduction)	3[b]	2–4	11	11
Infection	10?[c]			
Cogenital			2	2
Unknown	?		15	11

[a]These were included under "unknown" by Higginson and Muir [3].
[b]Much lower than number of cases because few skin cancers cause death.
[c]Considers hepatitis B virus and parasites which are not important factors in the United Kingdom.

has not been determined. Present views on predominant or avoidable causes are summarized in Table 5.

D. Individual Susceptibility

A small proportion of cancers are believed to be due to genetic or hereditary factors. For example, white skinned people of Celtic origin or individuals with xeroderma pigmentosa are unusually susceptible to a high frequency of skin cancer, as compared to black skinned people. There are probably many other unknown differences between people which may explain why, if two individuals are apparently exposed to the same exogenous risk, only one may develop cancer. Nonetheless, such situations in practice form only a small proportion of identified susceptibilities so that the identification of risks usually relates to external or other factors. It is believed that hepatitis B virus and aflatoxin may act together in causing cancer of the liver in Africa, but it is not yet established which factor is predominant. However, it appears that virus carriers are 200 times more sensitive than noncarriers.

IV. THE RISK OF CANCER

It is not possible to discuss here how epidemiological and experimental techniques are utilized to identify and measure the degree of risk associated with exposures to different carcinogens or carcinogenic risk factors. Among those epidemiological changes of greatest importance in identifying the possible role of carcinogenic stimuli are: (1) the differences in incidence of a specific cancer between communities which are ascribed to the environment, (2) changes in incidence following migration, whereby migrants develop the cancer patterns of their adopted country, and (3) changes in incidence over time. However, much of our present knowledge of specific avoidable causes and risks is derived from case-control or cohort studies in high risk populations, for example, population of individuals engaged in certain occupations, individuals who are smokers, drinkers, etc. Such studies permit determination not only of the background risk of cancer in a population, but also the added risk within a population subgroup due to a specific local environment.

Table 6 Percentage Chance of Developing Cancer by Age 75 in the United States (Connecticut Registry, 1968-1972)

Site	Cumulative risk[a]	
	Male	Female
Esophagus	0.69	0.14
Stomach	1.52	0.64
Colon and rectum	5.44	4.31
Lung	6.71	1.44
Breast	0.06	7.53
Prostate	4.07	—
Bladder	2.41	0.63
Brain	0.62	0.43
Leukemia	0.99	0.53
All sites	28.26	23.34

[a]Cumulative Risk is the probability that an individual will get cancer, apart from other illnesses, by age 75 years.
Source: Ref. [8].

In Table 6, the risk of developing cancer by age 75 is illustrated for the Connecticut population of the United States. The chance of a male getting cancer of the stomach is 1.5%, but nearly 7% for cancer of the lung. Altogether, a man has a chance of about 28% by the age of 75 to develop any type of cancer, the comparable figure for a woman being somewhat less. In evaluating occupational cancer, it is necessary to determine what added proportion of cancer is due to exposures in the workplace and the proportion due to other factors, since in all countries there appears to be a definite minimum risk of cancer. This requires that the background risk at a site be determined before the added risk of a suspected environmental factor, whether related to occupation, cultural habit, or lifestyle, can be determined.

Some of the highest rates in the world appear in Africa and Latin America. The rate for liver cancer in males in Bulawayo, Zimbabwe, for example, is very high and is probably related to aflatoxin poisoning. Conversely, in Latin America, the rate for cancer of the uterine cervix is exceedingly high.

A number of compilations have been made as to the lowest potential risks occurring in the world, and figures of approximately 10-20% of present rates within the United States are quoted. Many of these estimates do not take into account the role of lifestyle and dietary factors, which may be uncontrollable with present-day knowledge, and it is doubtful that such low rates will ever be attained in real life through avoidance of carcinogenic stimuli alone. Nonetheless, the low rates in a number of populations suggest that cancer incidence can be considerably reduced. Findings 30 years ago in South African blacks indicated that if the population did not smoke, their normal rate of cancer would be approximately a third of that in North America and Europe. Cancer rates among Mormons and Seventh Day Adventists are, for the men, approximately half, and for the women, about two-thirds to four-fifths that of the general U.S. population. This suggests that the impact of tobacco and alcohol is much less for women, and that other lifestyle factors such as diet and behavior are more important.

A. Cancer Patterns and Existing Carcinogenic Risk Factors

In recent years a number of calculations have been made to evaluate the proportion of cancers due to known causes. For methods of conducting such studies, reference should be made to the papers of Wynder and Gori [3], Higginson and Muir [4], and Doll and Peto [5]. These authors attribute approximately the same proportion of all cancers to specific risks. Tables 1-3 and 5 illustrate the major predominant causes believed responsible for 70-90% of cancers in humans in western industrial societies, discussed below in further depth.

1. Tobacco

This is by far the most important agent in human cancer, notably lung, that has been identified to date [7]. It is also believed to be a significant causal factor in cancers of the mouth, pharynx, bladder, pancreas, and kidney (Tables 4, 5). The evidence is conclusive that cigarette smoking is a direct cause of cancer, and further discussion on this point would appear worthless. Estimates of total cancers in the United States due to cigarette smoking vary between 30 and 40%. Doll and Peto [4] attributed to tobacco 43% of the 218,000 male and 15% of the 183,000 female cancer deaths in the United States. In addition to its direct effects, tobacco is also believed under certain circumstances to promote the effects of ionizing radiation, asbestos, and alcohol, and to potentiate their carcinogenic effects.

2. Alcohol

This is the most significant identified dietary factor related to cancer in humans in North America, Europe, and the Soviet Union. It is believed important in cancers of the liver, mouth, pharynx, larynx, and esophagus. Extensive studies have shown that the carcinogenic agent is probably ethanol, and not other compounds in alcoholic beverages. A synergistic effect of alcohol and tobacco has been shown in cancer of the esophagus. There is considerable evidence that the carcinogenic effect of even quite high consumption of alcoholic beverages is relatively small (two- to threefold) in nonsmokers for mouth cancer, but the incidence associated with high levels of alcohol and smoking may increase 80- to 150-fold, compared to nonsmoking individuals.

3. Occupational Exposures

Traditionally, observations in the workplace have played a major role in identifying powerful carcinogenic stimuli. Table 1 lists established occupational causes of cancer. There has been considerable argument as to the proportion of cancer due to occupation. The methods used in making such calculations are discussed by Higginson and Muir [3], Doll and Peto [4], and others. Most authors who have studied this problem have placed the proportion of cancers from 2–6% in males, and less than 2% in females in the sense of avoidable workplace risks. In view of the fact that exposures in the workplace have been changing rapidly in recent years, it is not clear to what extent these various estimates can be regarded with complete assurance as representative of future developments. There is a widespread belief that a large number of new carcinogens may have entered the environment in recent decades. However, preliminary investigation of a number of chemical companies suggests that the number of truly new formulas is much less than anticipated, the majority of new chemicals being mixtures of older compounds. This point requires more accurate clarification in order to develop more rational public health strategies in the future. Nonetheless, although the proportion of cancers due to chemical exposures may be relatively small in relation to the total burden of the disease, in a large country such as the United States this may translate into many thousands of cases. Furthermore, experience has shown that the cancers due to occupational exposures may be avoided by appropriate control of the hazardous exposures and are thus highly avoidable. Whereas hazardous situations are most likely to be identified in large industries where they can be adequately investigated, it is probable that the greatest burden of occupational, chemically induced cancer occurs in the relatively small industrial settings in the United States or in the developing countries. Unfortunately, such settings are precisely where unsatisfactory lifestyles are most likely to operate (for example, excessive smoking and drinking), and thus exact estimates of risk are difficult to calculate. As pointed out below, lifestyle is also now recognized as a factor of increasing importance in occupational differences.

4. Lifestyle Factors

In addition to smoking, alcohol, and occupation, other aspects of lifestyle may have a significant impact on tumors of the gastrointestinal and endocrine systems (Table 3). Of these, diet and behavior are the most important. Whereas a high proportion of all cancers are attributed by many authors to general aspects of lifestyle, including diet and behavior, the exact proportion is difficult to determine and requires further consideration. Recent developments in the laboratory in the field of cocarcinogenesis and the effects of agents affecting late-stage carcinogenesis have, however, suggested further possibilities in this context. There is considerable evidence that specific elements of diet may have their greatest impact in early childhood and possibly into midlife. This area has been inadequately explored. In recent years, however, the role of lifestyle has become of increasing importance in relation to certain workplace associated cancers. This has been most extensively studied in the United Kingdom, where it has been concluded that the majority of cancer variations within the workplace are related to the socioeconomic background of the population at risk, rather than to direct exposures within the workplace. This may be an important factor in the future in identifying healthy as opposed to unhealthy occupations. Unfortunately, few recent statistics within the United States are available to enable such evaluation. In South African black males, a much lower proportion of all cancers would be attributed to lifestyle, as aflatoxin in the diet is believed to be a factor in cancer of the liver, which comprises nearly 40% of all cancers.

5. Pollution

It is recognized that air, water, food, and so on, have contained contaminants and pollutants since man started using fire. Present controversy does not relate to heavy point source pollution as in an occupational setting, but rather to low-grade ambient pollution. The effects of the latter on cancer are difficult to detect, as the absolute risk from each pollutant is extremely low. Further, studies on air and water pollution have in general failed to demonstrate an effect of the total burden of pollutants present. Where pollutants have been identified in an industrial setting, it may be possible to make some numerical extrapolation downward from the known upper limit in order to theorize about risks of chronic exposure at levels of 100 to 1000 times lower. Previous attempts to do so have been largely concentrated on air pollution and the combustion of fossil fuels, probably acting in conjunction with cigarette smoking. In a 1977 symposium, it was concluded that combustion products are unlikely to account for more than 10% of the cases of lung cancer in smokers, and probably much less.

In regard to the role of pollutants in water, the only estimates we have at present are those by Doll and Peto that probably only less than 1% of all cancers relate to such factors, and again the correct figure is probably much less. It is not known to what extent such pollutants already present in the body may lead to a low level of background initiation in North America. Similar comments may be made about other industrial products in the general environment. The position in developing countries may be much worse and is only now becoming apparent.

6. Medical Therapy Related Cancers

A number of established human carcinogens have been used in medical practice, including ionizing radiation in cancer treatment, as well as estrogens and steroids in oral contraceptives (Table 2). Estrogens have been extensively used and have been effective in the treatment of postmenopausal symptoms and the prevention of osteoporosis. In one area of the United States, however, it is believed that they may have been responsible for a number of cases of endometrial cancer, and a significant drop in incidence has occurred in this tumor following cessation of their use. The use of estrogens in oral contraceptives has drawn the most interest, and despite many attempts, no evidence has been produced to suggest that these have had a significant effect on breast cancer. On the other hand, there is some evidence that they may inhibit endometrial and ovarian cancers.

7. Ionizing Radiation

Ionizing radiation has been utilized for treatment of cancer and is essential for diagnosis. However, in recent years there has been a marked reduction in exposures with improvement in technology. Doll and Peto [4] believe that continuation of present exposure levels could lead to the about 4500 fatal cases of cancer per year in the United States, but that much of this radiation has been used on individuals with life expectancies too small for any effect to be demonstrated. Their final estimate agrees with that of others that the rate is probably 1/2-1% of all cancers.

V. CONCLUSIONS

A review of existing cancer risks in the United States and Europe indicates that, by far, the major impact has been from such cultural habits as tobacco and alcohol. Secondly, diet and behavioral habits are believed significant, but individual factors have not been identified. Risk factors have been identified for approximately 50% of cancers in males and 15–20% of cancers in females in Europe and North America and thus offer a reasonable approach to control of avoidable causes.

REFERENCES

1. J. Clemmesen, *Statistical Studies in Malignant Neoplasams I. Review and Results*, Munksgaard, Copenhagen (1965).
2. E. L. Wynder and G. B. Gori, Contribution of the environment to cancer incidence: An epidemiologic exercise, *J. Natl. Cancer Inst., 58*:825-832 (1977).
3. J. Higginson and C. S. Muir, Environmental carcinogenesis: Misconceptions and limitations to cancer control, *J. Natl. Cancer Inst., 63*:1291-1298 (1979).
4. R. Doll and R. Peto, *The Causes of Cancer*, Oxford University Press, Oxford (1981).
5. J. F. Fraumeni Jr. (ed.), *Persons at High Risk of Cancer: An Approach to Cancer Etiology and Control*, Academic Press, New York (1975).
6. National Research Council, Assembly of Life Sciences, *Diet, Nutrition, and Cancer*, National Academy Press, Washington, D.C. (1982).
7. J. Cairns, *Cancer: Science and Society*, W. H. Freeman and Company, San Francisco (1978).
8. M. K. Stukonis, *Cancer Cumulative Risk*, IARC Internal Technical Report No. 79/004, International Agency for Research on Cancer, Lyon, France (1979).
9. E. C. Hammond and H. Seidman, Smoking and cancer in the United States, *Preventive Medicine, 9*:169-173 (1980).

2

REDUCING INDUSTRIAL CANCER: THE STRATEGIC AGENDA

William W. Lowrance*
Life Sciences and Public Policy Program
The Rockefeller University
New York, New York

*Formerly Special Assistant to U.S. Undersecretary of State for Security Assistance, Science, and Technology, and member of the faculties of Harvard and Stanford Universities, and Resident Fellow, National Academy of Sciences

I. "RISK"

"Risk" generally is taken to mean a factual estimate of the likelihood and severity of adverse effect—in the present case, the odds of incurring cancer. Societal or personal decisions about sources of risk are then understood to be appraisive, taking into account such considerations as benefits, costs, equities, and dynamics of decision, as well as risks.

However it may be expressed, "risk" is a compound of two notions: probability of harm and magnitude of harm. Thus, we assess the incidence (probability) of lower back injury (severity) at some manufacturing operation, or the chance of contracting angiosarcoma of the liver. Parallels are familiar from finance, as when we assess our expectations of gaining and losing various amounts from investments.

The estimation of health risks is in essence an empirical problem, even though it is surrounded by uncertainties. As is clear from the other chapters of this book, the facts about cancer incidence can be studied, and the carcinogenic properties of chemicals and radiation can be tested.

"Uncertainty" is not a good synonym for risk. As scientists use the term, uncertainty is a description of the precision and accuracy with which something is known or predicted from knowledge. One can easily imagine two hazardous situations (splinter in board versus tank of explosive solvent) about which one's risk prediction success is equivalently uncertain (being wrong, say, one time in a hundred predictions), but for which the risk stakes clearly are different.

There is no question but that empirical estimates of risk are value-conditioned (as all questioning is). Value orientation begins with the selection of the modes of hazard to be assessed (fatal harm or less serious illnesses, risk to workers or to workers' families or to neighborhood residents). Social value biases accrue as degrees of conservatism—choosing to err on the side of health precaution—are adopted in making estimates under scientific uncertainty.

After risks are estimated, decisions must be made about whether to bear the risks, or to reduce them by reducing their source or taking protective actions. Such decisions, often referred to as risk evaluation, are matters of personal and social value judgment. At issue may be whether a particular risk is "acceptable," or is similar to risks already accepted or to the risks of alternatives [1].

After *risk assessment* and *risk evaluation*, a third phase of action is taking practical steps to achieve *risk management*. As with managing any problem, this is value-laden: who to protect, how vigorously, at what cost.

A. Standard Approach to Decisions About Carcinogenic Risks

Schematized, decisions about environmental risks usually proceed as follows: (1) describe the existence of a hazard; (2) estimate human exposure to the hazard; (3) estimate effects expected for individuals from the exposure; (4) estimate prevalence, severity, and distribution of overall group or societal risk; (5) evaluate benefits and burdens associated with the source of hazard; compare the risks to other risks, especially the risks of alternatives to the present situation; appraise the practicalities of modifying the hazard; and then (6) decide whether to take action to reduce, redistribute, or compensate for the risks.

Although the process rarely is linear, all of these steps have to be worked through for an issue to become mature. It is important to cultivate such a conception of these decisions; otherwise they remain a perplexing muddle of contentions and uncertainties. These are the questions that have to be examined, whether the decisions are being made by industrial management, labor unions, government regulators, or independent evaluators.

B. Opportunities for Control

Only three basic types of control opportunity exist: (1) reduce the inherent hazard potential of the source of harm, as by changing chemical composition; (2) reduce exposure to the hazard; and (3) administer an antidote. For carcinogens no antidote or vaccine is known, so only the first two controls are possible: reduce the hazard or reduce exposure. Therefore, risk assessment must compare either different materials or different exposures (per person and per group of people potentially exposed).

II. THE CONTEXT OF INDUSTRIAL CANCER

A. Cancer Incidence

In this century cancer incidence in America has increased dramatically, in part because so many other causes of illness and death have been reduced. Also, the diagnosis of cancer has become more sensitive. Taken together, the dozens of different kinds of cancers add up to being the second leading cause of death in the United States (see Chapter 1). A heartening development is that recently the incidence of types of nonrespiratory cancer mortality has plateaued.

What proportion of the national cancer burden stems from workplace exposure to carcinogens? This is impossible to answer precisely. The most extensive cancer etiology analysis I know of, by Doll and Peto, estimated that about 4% of cancer deaths can be attributed to occupational causes. The authors acknowledged that their estimate is necessarily imprecise, but said that they thought it "unlikely to be out in either direction by more than a factor of two" [2].

B. Risk Reduction Accomplishments

During this century a great many occupational cancer risks have been reduced. In the last few decades exposure to ionizing radiation, such as x-rays, has been reduced many orders of magnitude. Asbestos exposure has been reduced substantially, and continues to be reduced further. Carcinogenic metals such as beryllium, nickel, cadmium, and chromium have been controlled. Although the chemicals still are handled in bulk quantities, a large variety of polycyclic hydrocarbons, amino-, nitro-, and chloroaromatics, vinyl chloride, and other chemicals have been "managed" so as to reduce exposure. So have large-volume chlorocarbon solvents such as carbon tetrachloride. Many possibly carcinogenic pesticides and dyes have been removed from the market. Where substitution has not been possible, processes in which suspect chemicals are handled have been isolated from worker contact.

For well known carcinogens, there now remain few instances in industry where an inspection team would find egregious violations of decent protection. Exceptions would include accidental (catastrophic, unintended) exposures, marginal sloppiness from careless waste disposal, neglect of personal hygiene, and violations of standard practice.

The largest sources of apprehension and controversy now are chemicals whose carcinogenic potential is not well understood or acknowledged.

C. Government Regulatory Frameworks

Major impetus for reduction of occupational cancer has been imparted by government, especially federal, regulation. The most powerful regulatory controls have been instituted since about 1970, in such laws as the Occupational Safety and Health Act, the Mine Safety and Health Act, the Toxic Substances Control Act, and amendments to the Atomic Energy Act.

A number of regulatory agencies, such as the Occupational Safety and Health Administration (OSHA), have been established to administer the regulatory provisions. Several research agencies, such as the National Institute of Occupational Safety and Health

(NIOSH, which is an agency of the Department of Health and Human Services), have been set up to perform research and assessment in support of, but in theory independent of, regulation.

These agencies' portfolios overlap. Their mandates are phrased differently, sometimes apparently inconsistently with each other. Often federal agencies come into conflict with state agencies, such as state occupational protection agencies. Especially in ill-defined and emergency situations, "environmental" bureaus (such as OSHA and the Environmental Protection Agency, EPA) may find themselves in jurisdictional tugs-of-war with "health" bureaus (such as the Centers for Disease Control, CDC), as is happening now with some toxic waste problems. And in dealing with hazards such as asbestos in shipyards, civilian bureaus may become hitched in uneasy tandem with their military counterparts.

Most of these agencies now have had over a decade to get established, try a variety of approaches, make some decisions, and learn from mistakes. The Congress, the courts, several different administrations, and a great many industry, labor, and other groups have, to put it blandly, provided feedback.

D. Industry Efforts

The only reliable generalization one can make about corporations' efforts to reduce hazard is that corporations differ widely among themselves in their attitudes and approaches.

But I believe it can be said that in the past decade substantial protections have been achieved by industry overall, that carcinogen research and control functions now are firmly integrated into most firms' operations, and that in general directors' and managers' commitments to protection have increased greatly.

Most sizeable firms have developed sophisticated quality control, toxicological testing, protective engineering, industrial hygiene, employee medical, and environmental monitoring capabilities. Some departments of the best firms consistently make and publish solid research contributions. There are, however, some large firms that have not developed these capabilities, and there are many smaller firms that have not. A large network of contract-research, testing and consulting firms, of varied reliability, have grown up to fill supplementary needs of firms (and government agencies).

Let us now dive from this background into the middle of current problems.

III. THE INDUSTRIAL CANCER "PROBLEM"

The "problem" comprises difficulties in all three major areas—carcinogenic risk assessment, risk evaluation, and risk management. It is compounded by the public's lack of technical understanding and by its abhorrence of the insidiousness and painfulness of cancer. Too, the cancer issue is, I suspect, in part a proxy for general distrust of industrial management.

A. Apprehension Overload

Some aspects of scientific progress entail a seeming paradox: as science improves, it raises awarenesses that raise public apprehensions. Analytic chemical techniques now can, for quite a few compounds in practice and countless others in theory (requiring only commitment of endeavor to work out the details), detect toxins in environmental media, food, or human tissues at a sensitivity of parts per billion—1/1,000,000,000 of the sample's weight! For a few compounds for which the effort was judged worth undertaking, analysis has reliably been conducted down a millionfold from that, to parts per quadrillion.

At such exquisite sensitivity it becomes evident that there is at least a little bit of everything in everything else. (Analytic chemists are constantly reminded of this in their never totally successful battle against contamination of solvents, glassware, and instruments.) This ability to detect, coupled with the inability precisely to assess human carcinogenicity at very low exposure, leads to the rueful conclusion I have often pointed to: About many chemicals we know enough to worry, but not enough to know *how much* to "worry," or how much protective action to invest.

Other factors also contribute to the public's apprehensiveness. Industrial chemicals continue to proliferate in variety and mode of application, as do new processes and products. And as we reduce exposure to materials that cause rare forms of cancer attributable to those particular carcinogenic materials—the asbestos that causes mesothelioma, the vinyl chloride that causes liver angiosarcoma— we are left confronting cancer types that seem to have many common possible causes. This raises the issue of small marginal elevations in incidence rates, a very difficult kind of causative problem to sort out.

B. Problems with Risk Assessment

As is widely conceded, the scientific assays currently available for assessing the carcinogenic potential of chemicals, dusts, and radiation (and alcohol consumption, psychological stress, and other lifestyle factors) are frustratingly inadequate. Being for the most part based on rodent assays, supplemented by inferences from inadvertent human exposures and by tests on bacteria and other primitive species, interpretation of these assays requires great inferential leaps: from bacteria and rodents to human beings, from relatively high exposures in the test animals to the relatively low exposures expeienced by workers. These problems have been discussed extensively elsewhere, so I will not review them here [3,4,5].

Concerned over the assessment approaches curently being used (and abused), in 1983 a National Research Council committee recommended to the Congress that a national Board on Risk Assessment Methods be established "to assess critically the evolving scientific basis of risk assessment and to make explicit the underlying assumptions and policy ramifications of the inference options in each component of the risk assessment process" and otherwise to critique agency guidelines and identify research needs [6]. Legislation has been introduced to accomplish this.

The predictive power of these tests will increase only as we accrue experience with more compounds and can discern associations between types of compounds and types of carcinogenic effects, and as we develop biochemical, genetic, and other fundamental knowledge of mechanism of action (see Chapters 3 and 4).

Complementation of laboratory testing comes from epidemiology—surveillance of worker populations over a long term to pick up indications of harm, and retrospective epidemiologic investigation of accidental and troubling exposures. Both are very hard to do. Problems stem from all the confounding factors of smoking, diet, and exposures to solvents, dusts, drugs, and so many other chemicals off the job. Problems arise in the question of "control" populations—who to compare the test group to? And in epidemiologic investigations there may arrive a moment when genuine suspicion exists about the hazard, but no conclusory evidence; this raises very difficult ethical managerial and regulatory decisions about disclosure and interim action.

C. Problems with Risk Evaluation

Nobody wants cancer. Everybody is willing to go to considerable expense to avoid it himself and to prevent it for others. But practical decisions about cancer risk still are difficult, for reasons that have to do with the following several "facts of life."

First, nothing—no material or activity—can be completely free of risk. In reducing one risk we often, in effect, just substitute other risks for it. Second, when we make personal or social decisions it is never only risks that we weigh, but also the benefits from the activities or circumstances that generate those risks, considerations of "fairness," and social power questions about *who decides what for whom.* And third, although human life may be beyond price, ventilation systems and electrostatic precipitators and medical surveillance programs most surely are not.

Thus industrial decisions have to do not with whether, say, leukemia is good or bad (I have never seen it taken as not-bad) but with whether, usually under great uncertainty about the facts, a financially important manufacturing process or product should be foregone, or modified at considerable expense, to reduce marginally an imputed cancer risk.

While there is true difficulty in appraising preventive investments, there are also complaints about regulatory decision frameworks. It is commonplace, and correct, to bemoan the fact that the various environmental regulatory laws phrase their mandates differently.

But we are going to have to admit that most of our legislated decision "frameworks" really are only versions of one framework. Regulation drafters often distinguish between "absolute no-risk" rules, benefit-risk balancing, cost-effectiveness, "best available technological control," protection "as low as is reasonably achievable," and the like. Really, however, in actual implementation these are distinctions without differences: "zero-risk" rules simply have been ignored when obeying them would be too costly for the benefit achieved; "available" control and "reasonable" achievability have been defined, pragmatically, by benefit-cost considerations; and although cost-effectiveness analysis does not estimate benefits, it assumes the benefits to be worth the effectively spent cost. I will return to this problem.

D. Problems with Risk Management

"Risk management," as I prefer to think of it, entails the entire range of actions undertaken to understand and control risks (this has sometimes been called "risk response"). This includes plant design, process design, procedures for handling materials from the moment they come through the plant gate until they leave (and then "following" them into use by industrial or consumer users), controlling all bulk waste and recycled materials, controlling fugitive dispersed wastes (vapors, dusts, smokes, soiled rags and clothing), monitoring personnel exposures, monitoring personnel health status, handling accidents, and performing all the research and analyses required to effect these risk management objectives.

Hardware always will need improving: better ventilators, filters, warning devices, and the like. But hardware is only part of the solution. Management and decision systems also are needed: better health surveillance systems, risk assessment protocols, waste-control provisions.

The risk management "problem" is partly technical. It is also economic and political and ethical. What criteria to use in choosing control strategies? How to prioritize risks for attention? How to reconcile corporate scientists' and managers' perceptions of risks with workers' and the general public's possibly different perceptions? How to handle the declared emergencies that arise when a material established in use becomes suspect as posing undue risk, either because scientific understanding changes or social values change?

IV. STRATEGIC AGENDA

I do not envision any panacea for reducing industrial cancer. Nor do I see any easy way of reducing public apprehensiveness. As was the case 50, 40, or 30 years ago in reducing industrial eye injuries (by changing design of countless processes and work situations, by providing eye guards and warning signs, by educating and cajoling and rewarding workers and supervisors, by reviewing eye-threatening accidents, by instituting routine ophthalmological surveillance and treatment, and so on), long hard work on a number of fronts will be necessary in reducing workplace cancer. The following are some recommendations for the agenda ("things that should be done").

A. Criteria for Carcinogen Assessment

The United States urgently needs a major, national, nonpartisan evaluation of the experiments and analyses used in assessing cancer risks, and of the criteria used in making regulatory decisions about them. Part of this could come from the Office of Science and Technology Policy review of chemical carcinogen policy published in May 1984 [3b] review that was begun several years ago but that has not, as of this writing (December 1983), been completed. Perhaps a study by a National Commission on Cancer Risk Evaluation could help, or a thorough, blue-ribbon review by the National Academy of Sciences. A number of case studies have been prepared, and others should be. Many reports are available as foundation material.

I cannot address the questions here, but they include: What has been the efficacy of "Ames-type" tests, rodent screening assays, and other such experimental approaches in predicting human carcinogenicity for chemicals we know from direct human evidence to be carcinogenic? How do the efficacies of the various designs of rodent and other mammalian assays compare with each other? How should various lesions be "counted"? How should statistical projections be made from animal to human experience? How should cancer "promoters" be regulated [7,8]? These questions are technical, but they embody many social value judgments, having to do especially with what degree of precaution to build into assessments.

Some of the most important questions simply are not empirical issues. What marginal reduction of the incidence of cancers should be judged "insignificant"? How should benefits and costs be brought into consideration? What to do when "we don't know" about a chemical? Much of this is appraisal and policy, not science.

The challenge is to institute assessment and evaluation approaches that are predictively valid, uniform, and applicable in consistent fashion in differing circumstances, but that at the same time allow flexible adaptation to new scientific understandings and to changes in social values.

B. Comparative Frameworks for Evaluation and Priority-Setting

Two methodological challenges to the agenda are to take more explicit approaches in dealing with all public health risks, and to develop comparative frameworks that will facilitate "sizing up" the threats relative to each other. Until we achieve these, organizations will continue to have to work piecemeal on problems, to be overloaded by demands, and to be distracted from working on undramatic but large ongoing risks by lesser risks presented as crises.

A striking example of explicitness and comparative evaluation is OSHA's 1983 standard for exposure to inorganic arsenic. In tightening the standard from 500 to $10 \mu g/m^3$, OSHA concluded "that inorganic arsenic is a carcinogen, that no safe level of exposure can be demonstrated, and that $10 \mu g/m^3$ is the lowest possible level to which employee exposure could be controlled." Further,

> The level of risk from working a lifetime of exposure at $10 \mu g/m^3$ is estimated at approximately 8 excess lung cancer

deaths per 1000 employees. OSHA believes that this level of risk does not appear to be insignificant. It is below risk levels in high risk occupations but it is above risk levels in occupations with average levels of risk.

Surely this rationale is commendable (regardless of whether the particular numbers adopted survive current dispute) [9].

Similar reasoning is being applied by other agencies. For instance, the EPA has said, in regulating N-nitroso pesticides, that "Solely for the purpose of establishing priorities, the 1×10^{-6} (one-in-a-million) level appears from a policy perspective to be a reasonable criteria (sic) to help separate high risk (and high resource) situations from low risk problems [10]."

This naturally leads to the idea of "triage," or separating threats into three categories: those trivially or insignificantly low, those intolerably high, and those worth devoting effort on to study, debate, and try to reduce. The Food and Drug Administration has ruled the risks of several hair dyes and food colorings "insignificant" compared to other hazards. OSHA in the past has developed carcinogen priority lists, based on preliminary evaluations. The EPA has ranked the nation's toxic waste sites as to public health menace and emergency character.

Several schemes for ranking carcinogenic potency of chemicals have been proposed. One of the most discussed is that used by the International Agency for Research on Cancer, which grades the "sufficiency of evidence" of carcinogenic risk for chemicals [11]. Robert Squire has proposed a scheme that is more sensitive to distinctions based on mechanistic understanding [12]. Neither of these, however, solves the risk assessment problem, because neither takes into account such factors as individual exposure, prevalence of that exposure through society, or benefits derived from the source of the risk.

Deisler has proposed use of risk ceilings (limits of acceptability) related to national cancer risk-reduction goals; those goals would be established by legislation, following broad national debate [13]. Although such a goal has not been established, it could be deliberated on as part of the national commission effort I am recommending.

Such rationalization is being achieved, in essence, albeit slowly and in piecemeal fashion, as present regulations are "tuned" up and down within the 10^{-3}–10^{-7} lifetime cancer risk range. Most of the current regulatory debates in Washington have to do with marginal risk differences (for exposure, or for alternative chemicals) of about one order of magnitude; this is the case, for example, with benzene, formaldehyde, and many pesticides. The OSHA arsenic standard just mentioned is an exception.

Recently a British Royal Society study group reasoned as follows [14]:

> If the average expectation of life is 70–75 years, then the imposition of a continuing annual risk of death to the individual of 10^{-2} seems unacceptable. At 10^{-3} it may not be totally unacceptable if the individual knows of the situation, enjoys some commensurate benefit, and everything reasonable has been done to reduce the risk. At the other extreme, there are levels of assumed annual risk so low that the manager or regulator can regard them as trivial.

Again, a problem for all such approaches is to factor in considerations of benefit and cost. A 10^{-4} risk associated with a frivolous product may be tolerated far less willingly than the same risk incurred from a societally important process or product.

C. Risk Management Opportunity Analysis

An important source of guidance that deserves developing is what I call risk management opportunity analysis: estimating the information gains and control gains that can be expected from various contemplated research or control strategies. Often it is possible, even with imprecise input numbers, to go through a very illuminating analysis of prospects. A team at Decision Focus Incorporated compared the cancer reduction effectiveness that can be expected from various physical controls (at estimated costs) of the dry cleaning fluid perchloroethylene [15]. Weinstein has performed an analysis of the cancer reduction "payoff" of large-scale rodent carcinogen assays (and compared it to the possible returns from investigation and beta-carotene as a dietary cancer prevention agent) [16,17]. Decision analysis of this kind holds considerable promise and should be considered, where possible, by administrators when strategies are being developed [18].

D. Other Initiatives

1. Dealing Forcibly with "Leftover" Chemical Hazards

It is important both for reducing risk and for allaying public fears that firms deal forthrightly and forcibly with such hazards as asbestos, chemical waste, and other problems left over from earlier eras. Some product lines may even have to be abandoned.

In part this is an adjustment to changes in social values; like all such adjustments, it is not easy. My hope is that the nation has become so much more sophisticated about anticipating and minimizing risks that it will, in the run of the next decades, be very unlikely to let a hazard develop to the dimensions of, say, the asbestos legacy we now are coping with. Sermon: Get past the current big ones, redress the damages as fully as possible, then guard against letting those kinds of risks develop again. And in the process, bolster public confidence.

2. Improvement of Social Mechanisms for Gathering, Filtering, and Certifying Scientific Information, and for Moderating Technicosocial Disputes

The improvements in peer review and outside advisory panel review of recent years obviously should be encouraged. So should such new institutions as the Chemical Industry Institute of Toxicology, and such broad-based consensus development projects as the formaldehyde conference convened by the National Center for Toxicological Research in October 1983.

Central coordinated worker registries and associated follow-up, such as that established by the National Institute for Occupational Safety and Health for soft-tissue sarcomas, can provide efficient research bases and can focus technical controversy.

William Ruckelshaus, the Administrator of EPA, has made the following plea: "Scientists must be willing to take a larger role in explaining the risks to the public—including the uncertainties inherent in any risk assessment. Shouldering this burden is the responsibility of all scientists, not just those with a particular policy end in mind" [19]. It is important to "fill the middle" in disputes.

3. Education and Sensitization

There is a serious need to inform journalists, the general public, and business, labor, and government officials of all these matters.

More than anything else, what is needed is broad comprehension of the *complexion* of the issues as social problems—what is being asked, what is being hassled over, what is at stake, how these issues dovetail with other social issues.

Firms and unions can help by sensitizing not only their operations and issues managers, but their top officials, lawyers, and public spokesmen. Seminars in community colleges can help, as can seminars for journalists. Few business or medical schools address these problems firmly, and they should. There is also a need to sensitize industrial technical personnel as they move up from laboratories or design rooms into management positions.

An important corrective to the despair that tends to creep into this arena is to inculcate a view of risk management efforts as societal investments—investments that yield returns in health costs saved, disruptions reduced, productivity enhanced, and goodwill maintained [20].

REFERENCES

1. W. W. Lowrance, Choosing our pleasures and our poisons: Risk assessment for the 1980's, in *Science, Technology, and the Issues of the Eighties: Policy Outlook* (A. H. Teich and R. Thornton, eds.), Westview Press, Boulder, CO, 1982.
2. R. Doll and R. Peto, *The Causes of Cancer*, Oxford University Press, Oxford, 1981.
3. U.S. Congress, Office of Technology Assessment, *Assessment of Technologies for Determining Cancer Risk from the Environment*, U.S. Government Printing Office, Washington, D.C., 1981.
4. Task Force of Past Presidents of the Society of Toxicology, Animal data in hazard evaluation: Paths and pitfalls, in *Fundamental and Applied Toxicology*, 2:101 (1982).

5. U.S. Office of Science and Technology Policy, Chemical carcinogens, *Fed. Reg., 49*, 21,594 (May 22, 1984).

6. National Research Council, Committee on the Institutional Means for Assessment of Risk to Public Health, *Risk Assessment in the Federal Government: Managing the Process*, National Academy Press, Washington, D.C., 1983.

7. Subcommittee on Department Operations, Research, and Foreign Agriculture, of the Committee on Agriculture, U.S. House of Representatives, Regulation of Pesticides, 1983.

8. Subcommittee on Commerce, Transportation, and Tourism of the Committee on Energy and Commerce, U.S. House of Representatives, *Hearings on Cancer Policy and the Control of Carcinogens in the Environment*, March 17, 1983.

9. U.S. Occupational Safety and Health Administration (OSHA), Occupational exposure to inorganic arsenic, *Fed. Reg., 48*:1867 (January 14, 1983).

10. U.S. Environmental Protection Agency (EPA), Pesticides contaminated with N-nitroso compounds: Proposed policy, *Fed. Reg., 45*:42,854 (June 25, 1980).

11. International Agency for Research on Cancer, *The Evaluation of the Carcinogenic Risk of Chemicals to Humans*, Monograph *22*, Lyon, France, 1980.

12. R. A. Squire, Ranking animal carcinogens: A proposed regulatory approach, *Science, 241*:877 (1981).

13. P. F. Deisler, Jr., Dealing with industrial health risks: A stepwise goal-oriented approach, in *Risk in the Technological Society* (C. Hohenemser and J. X. Kasperson, eds.), Westview Press, Boulder, CO, 1982.

14. Royal Society Study Group on Risk, *Risk Assessment*, The Royal Society, London, 1983, p. 17.

15. G. L. Campbell, D. Cohan, and D. W. North, *The Application of Decision Analysis to Toxic Substances: Proposed Methodology and Two Case Studies*, A report to the U.S. Environmental Protection Agency, National Technical Information Service, #PB82-249-103, Washington, D.C., 1982.

16. M. C. Weinstein, Cost-effective priorities for cancer prevention, *Science, 221*:17, (1983).

17. J. D. Graham and J. W. Vaupel, Value of a life: What difference does it make?, *Risk Analysis, 1*:89 (1981).

18. National Research Council, Steering Committee on Identification of Toxic and Potentially Toxic Chemicals for Consideration by the Na-

tional Toxicology Program, *Strategies to Determine Needs and Priorities for Toxicity Testing*, Vol. 1, National Academy Press, Washington, D.C., 1981.

19. W. D. Ruckelshaus, Science, risk, and public policy, *Science, 221*:1026 (1983).

20. W. W. Lowrance, Improved science, heightened societal aspirations, and the agenda for 'risk' decision making, in *Risk in Society* (A. J. Jouhar, ed.), John Libbey & Company Limited, London, 1983.

3

THE USES OF TOXICOLOGY AND EPIDEMIOLOGY IN IDENTIFYING AND ASSESSING CARCINOGENIC RISKS

Robert A. Neal and James E. Gibson
Chemical Industry Institute of Toxicology
Research Triangle Park, North Carolina

39

I. INTRODUCTION

Some percentage of cancer in man results from exposure to carcinogenic chemicals, both natural and manmade (see Chapter 1). Some portion of this chemically induced cancer may be prevented by reducing or eliminating exposure. Therefore, given the public concern with cancers, considerable scientific and regulatory attention has centered on efforts to identify actual or potential human carcinogens present in human environments or which may be introduced by certain industrial practices or technological changes.

The purpose of this chapter is to examine the techniques and procedures currently available for identifying those chemical and physical factors in the industrial environment which are carcinogenic or potentially carcinogenic to humans. Further, the methods used to assess or predict the risk associated with low-dose exposure of humans to carcinogenic chemicals is reviewed.

II. METHODS FOR ASSESSING CARCINOGENICITY

The principal techniques available are epidemiology, so-called "short-term" tests, animal bioassays, and structure-activity relationships. Each technique has its strengths and limitations.

A. Epidemiology

Epidemiology plays an important role in identifying carcinogenic chemicals in an industrial environment. It is also useful in identifying exposures which may be associated with an increased incidence of cancer, although the agent or agents responsible for the increased incidences may often not be identified.

In applying epidemiological methods to the detection of cancer in industrial populations, a positive relationship is based on the statistical significance of the data. However, it is important to remember that a positive statistical association does not necessarily mean that a cause-effect relationship has been established. Negative epidemiological studies are also useful in that they help define the upper limit of human cancer risk.

Those industrial situations where chemicals have been shown by epidemiological studies to be causally related to the occurrence of cancer in humans have been the result of high exposure of relatively small population groups. Therefore, as noted by Tomatis [1], the identification of human carcinogens has occurred under conditions of exposure similar to those used in experimental carcinogenesis. That is, conditions where a limited number of experimental animals are exposed to high levels of the chemical or mixture of chemicals in order to increase the sensitivity of the animal surrogates.

The first uses of epidemiology to identify an occupational cancer hazard were the observations of Pott in 1775 [2]. Pott correctly concluded that scrotal cancer in chimney sweeps was caused by exposure to soot. An example of the recent use of epidemiological evidence to establish cancer causality with chemical exposure is the increase in the incidence of angiosarcoma of the liver of vinyl chloride-exposed workers [3]. The International Agency for Research on Cancer (IARC) has identified 16 chemicals and industrial processes, in addition to soot and vinyl chloride, for which there is sufficient epidemiological evidence to indicate a causal relationship between exposure and an increased cancer incidence in humans [4]. The IARC identified 18 additional chemicals for which the epidemiologic evidence was more limited but which suggested these chemicals were *probably* carcinogenic for humans [4].

Thus, epidemiology is indeed an important technique in the identification of human carcinogens. However, there are major limitations to it. Epidemiology obviously cannot be used to assess the potential carcinogenicity of chemicals to which human exposure is anticipated. Because most human exposures are to such low levels as to preclude the direct measurement of risk, negative results do not necessarily demonstrate the absence of hazard because of the insensitivity of epidemiological methods in detecting increases in cancer incidences. Although an increase in the incidence of a rare human cancer may be detected using epidemiology, an increase in common cancers such as cancer of the lung, breast, or colon will not likely be detected except in the case of high incidence of the disease. The long latency period between first exposure to a carcinogenic chemical or physical factor and the clinical detection of the tumor limits the usefulness of epidemiology. Suitable unexposed control groups are sometimes difficult to obtain if exposure to the chemical is widespread. Finally, large-scale epidemiological studies, particularly cohort studies, are very expensive.

In spite of these limitations, epidemiology is a valuable technique. It is the only method currently available which provides direct evidence of the presence or absence of *human* cancer risks. Finally, the results of epidemiological studies, in combination with the results from animal oncogenicity studies, and studies using various techniques for measuring the ability of the chemicals to alter the structure of DNA in plant and animal cells, allow a more accurate determination of the potential cancer risk to humans than can be arrived at by evaluating the results of each of the various techniques separately.

B. Short-Term Tests

Substantial evidence indicates that one step in carcinogenesis is damage to or mutation of the DNA. Many bacterial and mammalian cell culture assays can detect such alterations induced by chemicals. Because there is some correlation between the activity of chemicals in these assays and the carcinogenic activity of these chemicals in rodents, they have been termed "short-term" tests for potential carcinogenicity. Substantial progress has been made in the development of these assays so that one can now measure chemically induced alteration of DNA in bacteria, insects, mammalian cells in culture, human cells in culture and, in some cases, in cells from living animals exposed to these chemicals. The short-term tests currently available can be broadly classified into three major groups: those that detect gene mutations and chromosome aberrations, those that are capable of detecting transformation of mammalian cells in vitro, and those that measure interactions of chemicals with critical molecules (primarily DNA).

It is now well accepted that chemically induced increases in cancer incidence in mammals is a multistage process. These various stages in the carcinogenic process include, at a minimum, initiation, promotion, and progression. It is also clear that there are many different mechanisms by which chemicals can induce cancer. For example, chemicals may cause a somatic mutation, alter hormonal balance, cause increased cell turnover, or hyperplasia of certain cell types, all of which may result in an increase in cancer incidence. Unquestionably, there are additional biological factors which may be altered by chemicals resulting in an increase in cancer incidence. This diversity in the etiology of cancer and the multistage nature of the process has important implications relative to the development and utilization of short-term tests for the detection of potential human carcinogens. Thus, there is a need for short-term tests that measure the various events that may be responsible for induction of cancer in humans (e.g., initiation, promotion, progression, hyperplasia, hormonal imbalance, etc.). Cairns [5] has recently suggested that spontaneous or chemically induced chromosome rearrangements may present a more critical event in the induction of human cancer than gene mutations. Thus, there is also a need for short-term tests which can reliably detect those chromosome rearrangements which may be important in the induction of cancer. Unless or until short-term tests are available to measure all the various biological events which are important in cancer induction in humans and experimental animals, their usefulness will be limited. For example, the majority of the short-term tests currently available are based on the hypothesis that mutation or damage to DNA is the critical event in the induction of cancer in humans. However, several studies have shown that the various short-term tests which detect mutation of or damage to DNA are unable to identify a substantial number of chemicals known to be carcinogenic in humans and experimental animals.

One of the difficulties in using the results of short-term tests to identify chemicals potentially carcinogenic to humans and experimental animals is differences in the metabolic disposition of the chemicals in the in vitro short-term tests as compared to the whole animal. Many of these short-term systems either lack or have much lower levels of those enzymes and enzyme systems present in

intact animals which are known to extensively metabolize xeno-
biotic chemicals to both active and inactive carcinogenic metabolites. An external source of these enzymes and enzyme systems is
often provided in short-term tests. However, these exogenous enzyme sources may not accurately reflect the metabolism which occurs in vivo. Therefore, there is considerable research activity currently underway to develop and validate in vivo methods in experimental animals for measuring biological processes believed to be
involved in the induction of cancer in humans. Tests in intact experimental animals allow the chemicals under study to be subjected to the same absorption, distribution, metabolism, and excretion processes as is generally the case in humans. Moreover, in
the intact animal, any alterations in biological processes involved
in the induction of cancer may be subject to reversal or repair.
These same processes of reversal or repair would likely be operative in humans exposed to the chemicals in question.

Published in the preamble to the recent IARC monographs is
an assessment of the utility of short-term tests in determining the
potential carcinogenicity of chemicals to humans or experimental
animals [6]. This preamble states that because the mechanisms of
carcinogenesis are incompletely understood, the results of the
short-term tests "should not be used by themselves to conclude
whether or not an agent is carcinogenic." The preamble also concludes that the results of short-term tests should not be used to
predict the carcinogenic potency of a chemical in experimental
animals and humans.

The IARC monographs [6] also describe a classification scheme
for the validity of the results obtained with a chemical in short-
term tests; it is based on the strength of the evidence that a chemical displays activity in these tests. The first category is *sufficient
evidence*. Sufficient evidence of activity is judged to have been
shown "when there were a total of at least three positive results in
at least two of three test systems measuring DNA damage, mutagenicity, or chromosomal anomalies." *Limited evidence* is shown
"when there were at least two positive results, either for different
endpoints or in systems representing two levels of biological
complexity." *Inadequate evidence* is available "when there were

too few data for an adequate evaluation or when there were con-
tradictory data." *No evidence* is described as that condition "when
there were many negative results from a variety of short-term tests
with different endpoints, and at different levels of biological
complexity."

In summary, there are substantial limitations to the use of data
from the short-term tests currently available in cancer risk assessment. Perhaps the most severe limitation is the lack of quantitative relationships between the results of short-term tests and cancer incidence in experimental animals [7-11]. However, short-
term tests can be useful in the assay of a series of chemicals or
mixtures of chemicals which cannot, for various reasons, all be
tested in experimental animals for their potential to be carcinogenic in humans. Here, they can be useful in prioritizing chemicals
for testing in experimental animals. They can also be useful in providing information about industrial treatment or process changes
which may eliminate or reduce the levels of potential human carcinogens. Finally, short-term tests carried out in conjunction with
animal tests and/or epidemiological studies can be helpful in arriving at a better understanding of the biological mechanisms by
which a particular chemical or chemical mixture is causing an increase in cancer incidence in experimental animals or humans and,
consequently, a better estimate of the potential risk to humans
from exposure to that chemical or chemical mixture.

C. Animal Bioassays

The results of animal bioassays, conducted largely in rodents, have
been and will continue to be the major source of data for estimating human risk from exposure to potentially carcinogenic
chemicals in the industrial environment. The essence of the animal
bioassay for carcinogenicity is to observe test animals for a major
portion of their life span for the appearance of tumors resulting
from exposure to various doses of a chemical or chemical mixture.

Because of cost and availability, rats and mice are almost exclusively used to assess the potential carcinogenicity of chemicals
to humans. Although there are exceptions, many of the neoplasms

produced by chemicals in rats and mice have similar morphological and behavioral characteristics to those in man. Also, with some exceptions, these animals are metabolically and anatomically similar to man. Since the production of cancer from exposure to chemicals is often related to metabolism of the chemical to a reactive intermediate, the metabolic similarity is of extreme importance. It is also important to note that the rodent species used in testing are subject to many of the diseases which man suffers.

One method for judging the adequacy of the animal bioassay to accurately identify potential human carcinogens is to examine those chemicals known to be carcinogenic in humans for their ability to cause cancer in animal models. Of the 18 chemicals or industrial processes known to be carcinogenic in humans [4], 14 have been examined for their ability to cause cancer in experimental animals. Of these 14 chemicals, ten have produced cancer in experimental animals. Of the four remaining compounds, arsenic has not produced tumors in any animal model. Benzene has not yet been shown to produce a statistically significant increase in tumors in rats or mice by inhalation, the most appropriate route. However, an increase in tumors is produced in experimental animals if benzene is administered by gavage. Convincing evidence of carcinogenicity has not yet been shown in animals administered mustard gas or chlornaphazine. Of the 18 chemicals or industrial processes judged to be *probably* carcinogenic for humans [4], 16 have been shown to produce cancer in experimental animals. Limited data are available on the carcinogenicity of the remaining compounds, auramine and oxymetholone. Thus there is a reasonable, although not complete, qualitative correlation between the ability of chemicals to cause cancer in humans and experimental animals. In these comparisons, the target organ for carcinogenicity was the same for experimental animals and humans in about 80% of the cases. In this regard, similar target organs were seen more often if the routes of exposure of humans and the experimental animals were the same. The most prominent exception in the correlation of target organs in experimental animals and humans occurred with compounds which produced bladder tumors in humans.

The ability of the rodent bioassays to detect potential human carcinogens has also been examined in another way. Recently, Purchase [12], examined data on 250 chemicals which have been tested for carcinogenicity in both rats and mice. Of the 126 chemicals found to be positive for cancer in rats, only 87% were positive for cancer in mice. Of the 119 chemicals found to be negative for cancer in the rat, only 82% were negative for the mouse. Conversely, of the 130 chemicals found to be positive for cancer in the mouse, only 84% were positive for cancer in the rat. Of the 115 chemicals which were found to be negative for cancer in the mouse, only 85% were negative for cancer in the rat. These data allow a determination of how accurately the mouse can predict for the ability of chemicals to cause cancer in the rat and vice versa. Thus, the rat as a predictor of chemically induced cancer in the mouse has a specificity of about 85%. The mouse as a predictor of cancer in the rat has a specificity of about 82%. It is reasonable to assume that the ability of the rat or mouse to predict for the potential or lack of potential of a chemical to cause cancer in man is no better than their ability to predict for cancer in each other. Adamson and Sieber have recently published a review of their studies of the carcinogenicity in nonhuman primates of eight model rodent carcinogens [13]. With the exception of urethane, none of these model compounds has yet induced tumors in Old World monkeys even after prolonged periods of administration and observation. Thus, the rodent as a model for detecting potential human carcinogens has an implied degree of unreliability. There is even greater uncertainty regarding the validity of using dose-response data from studies in laboratory rodents for quantitative evaluation of cancer risk in humans.

Of the various schemes for categorizing the results of animal studies for evidence that the chemical or chemical mixture is an animal carcinogen, the IARC classification [4] is most widely accepted by the informed scientific community. Listed below are the five IARC classifications.

1. *Sufficient evidence* of carcinogenicity indicates that there is an increased incidence of malignant tumors: (a) in multiple species or strains; or (b) in multiple experiments (preferably with differ-

ent routes of administration or using different dose levels); or (c) to an unusual degree with regard to incidence, site or type of tumor, or age at onset. Additional evidence may be provided by data concerning dose-response effects, as well as information on mutagenicity or chemical structure.

2. *Limited evidence* of carcinogenicity means that the data suggest a carcinogenic effect but are limited because: (a) the studies involve a single species, strain, or experiment; or (b) the experiments are restricted by inadequate dosage levels, inadequate duration of exposure to the agent, inadequate period of follow-up, poor survival, too few animals, or inadequate reporting; or (c) the neoplasms produced often occur spontaneously or are difficult to classify as malignant by histological criteria alone (e.g., lung and liver tumors in mice).

3. *Inadequate evidence* indicates that because of major qualitative or quantitative limitations, the studies cannot be interpreted as showing either the presence or absence of a carcinogenic effect.

4. *Negative evidence* means that within the limits of the tests used, the chemical is not carcinogenic. The number of negative studies is small since, in general, studies that show no effect are less likely to be published than those suggesting carcinogenicity.

5. *No data* indicates that data were not available to the working group.

The categories *sufficient evidence* and *limited evidence* refer only to the strength of the experimental evidence that these chemicals are (or are not) carcinogenic and not to the extent of their carcinogenic activity. The classification for any chemical may change as new information becomes available.

The IARC has also stated its position concerning the evaluation of the results of carcinogenicity studies conducted in experimental animals [14]. In this document it is stated that in the absence of adequate data in humans it is reasonable, for practical purposes, to regard chemicals for which there is *sufficient evidence* of carcinogenicity in animals as if they presented a *carcinogenic risk* for humans. Inherent in this statement is the implication that a correlation between carcinogenicity in animals and possible human risk cannot be made on a scientific basis. Rather, the statement is a pragmatic one, made with the intent of assisting regulatory agencies in making decisions related to the control of potentially carcinogenic substances.

D. Important Elements of Animal Bioassays

Although there are variations in various animal bioassays designed to adequately test for the carcinogenicity of chemicals, they all contain some basic elements. These include that the chemical should be examined in both sexes of at least two species. As noted previously, rats and mice are usually the species used. At least two doses should be administered. The minimum number of animals of each sex at each dose is usually 50. A suitable control group of the same size should be included. The exposure should start shortly after weaning and continue for approximately 24 months. The animals should be closely monitored throughout the study and gross and histopathological examination conducted on those animals which die during the study and on at least the high dose and controls at the termination of the study. Additional details of the conduct of chronic bioassays are described in various published guidelines [15,16].

Attention to certain key elements of the basic animal chronic bioassays can improve the usefulness of the data in estimating human cancer risk. Among these are dose selection and route of exposure. In addition, studies of the biotransformation of the chemical and studies of the biological mechanisms of the carcinogenic effect seen with that chemical can be of considerable value in determining the applicability of the results of the animal carcinogenic bioassay to humans.

1. Dose, Toxicokinetics, Metabolism

There are a number of factors which must be considered in the selection of doses for the study of the potential of a chemical (with due regard to its impurities) or mixture of chemicals to cause cancer in experimental animals. One of these is the number of doses to be administered. If the purpose of the study is simply to determine if the compound or mixture of compounds has the capacity to cause cancer in one or more species of experimental animals, then one carefully selected dose may be sufficient. If the purpose of the study is both to determine the capacity of the chemical to cause cancer in one or more species as well as to assess the shape of the dose-response curve in those species for the purpose of human risk assessment, then more than one dose must be administered. The question is, how many doses should be administered to provide ample data for risk assessment? There is a general consensus that at least three dose levels should be used in addition to the concurrent control group. These doses should be chosen so as to give a gradation of response.

When mixed in the diet, a compound may change the nutritional quality of the diet. It may do this by changing the nutritional balance of the diet, by affecting intestinal absorption of nutrients either directly or by way of inducing diarrhea, decrease the palatability of the diet, induce anorexia, or reduce the availability of some micronutrients.

The effect of diet composition such as the relative fat content, protein-calorie ratio, or decreased calorie intake on tumor incidence in experimental animals is well known. If a nutritional effect of the compound under study is suspected based on the results of the subchronic study, the nature of these effects should be determined and the appropriate adjustments made, including an adjustment of doses, before the carcinogenicity study is begun.

It is desirable that the highest dosage level administered in the animal bioassay for carcinogenicity not exceed the ability of the animal species under study to excrete it in a manner which is approximately the same as at lower dosages. In addition, the high dose should not lead to the formation of metabolites which are not seen at the lower dosages which are more nearly equivalent to those to which humans will be exposed. A change in manner of excretion with increasing dose can be detected by an abrupt change in the relationship between the plasma concentration of the substance and the administered dose. A qualitative change in metabolism with increasing dose can be detected by identifying the metabolites present in various tissue and excretion products of the animals. Dosages above and below those at which one sees changes in the mechanism of excretion or metabolism should be administered in the chronic study. This use of toxicokinetic and metabolic data in setting the doses will help in the interpretation of the results of the bioassay. Toxicokinetic studies will also allow the determination of those compounds with long half-lives of excretion, important information in setting the highest dosage in the chronic study. Finally, evidence gained from metabolism studies which indicates the formation of chemically reactive metabolites of the compounds under study will also be of value in interpreting the results of the chronic study.

Ideally, studies of subchronic toxicity, toxicokinetics, and metabolism and other considerations as noted previously, should be used in setting the high dose to be administered in the chronic study. Unfortunately, the result of a subchronic toxicity study is often the only data available for this purpose. In that case, the high dose should elicit some minimal signs of toxicity unrelated to any cancer which may develop without altering the normal life span. There is some disagreement in the scientific community on what degree of minimal toxicity should be seen. Most agreement seems to center on a significant difference in weight gain or final body weight in the high-dose animals as compared to controls, but not to exceed 10%. However, the figure of 10% should not be considered to have some special scientific validity.

2. Route of Administration

The major routes of administration of compounds in carcinogenicity studies are oral, mixed in the diet or drinking water, by gastric intubation, or via inhalation. Less common are dermal application, subcutaneous or intraperitoneal injection, intramuscular or intravenous injection, intranasal or intrapulmonary placement or implantation. As a general rule, the compound under study should be administered by the route that most closely duplicates the one by which human exposure occurs or may occur. There are instances where humans may be exposed to a compound by more than one route, for example, by both inhalation and dermal absorption. In these cases the question is, which should be the route of administration? Common sense dictates that, assuming equal exposure by both routes, the compound should be administered by the route judged to pose the greatest potential risk. In the case where one route of exposure predominates over another, the predominant route should be considered as the most appropriate in the animal studies.

Because of certain physical or chemical properties of the chemical under study, or the lack of appropriate facilities for exposure of the experimental animals by the most appropriate route, gastric intubation is used. This method of exposure has several limitations. There may be some mortality during the intubation process. If a vegetable oil solvent is used, the nutritional balance of the diet may be changed and biological effects may occur that compromise the interpretation of the study. Artificially higher tissue levels of the compound under study may be obtained when the compound is administered by gastric intubation as compared to inhalation or incorporation into drinking water or diet, leading to acute or subacute toxicity or, perhaps, to chronic toxicity which would not be seen if the compound were administered by the more appropriate route. In substituting gastric intubation for dietary, dermal or inhalation exposure, consideration should be given in setting the highest dose to be administered by gastric intubation, to the peak tissue concentrations of the compound seen when a maximum tolerated dose is administered by the most appropriate route.

3. Species Selection

As noted previously, there are some qualitative differences in the response of various species to carcinogenic chemicals. There are a number of factors responsible for these differences; included among these are anatomic, physiologic, or biochemical differences, differences in metabolism, differences in the sensitivity of receptors, and differences in rats and routes of excretion. Where data from human exposure to the compound of interest are available or studies with human tissues have been carried out, these data should be taken into account in selecting the best species for use in a chronic study.

4. Mechanisms of Toxicity

Knowledge of the mechanisms of the carcinogenic effects of chemicals can be extremely useful in assessing the reliability of the rodent models as predictors of carcinogenic effects in humans. Short-term tests that examine possible mechanisms of carcinogenesis, including evidence for and against alteration of DNA structure, can also provide valuable information. However, the most valuable information for determining the reliability of a particular rodent model in predicting human cancer would be comparative studies of the toxicokinetics, metabolism, and genotoxicity of the compound in both humans and rodents. In these studies, results from humans occupationally—and accidentally—exposed to the compound could be used where they can ethically be obtained. If such results are not available, experimental studies with human tissues obtained at autopsy or surgery will provide valuable information, especially in comparison with identical studies in rodent tissues. After a substantial body of information has been accumulated comparing toxicokinetics, metabolism, genotoxicity, and other biological effects of carcinogenic chemicals in humans and rodent models, a more accurate assessment of the predictability of our rodent models for chemically induced cancer in man can be made.

The term genetic carcinogen is used to describe a compound which directly interacts with the genetic material and causes an irreversible change in the structure of DNA that leads to a cell with the potential to grow and produce a tumor. The term epigenetic carcinogen refers to compounds that increase the tumor incidence in experimental animals and humans indirectly by some mechanism other than a direct irreversible change in the structure of the DNA of the cells in question.

Some genetic carcinogens cause cancer by producing an irreversible change in the genetic information encoded in the DNA of somatic cells, but require the action of another chemical or chemicals for the cells to rapidly divide and form a tumor. Other compounds may cause an increase in neoplasia because they are complete carcinogens. That is, they can cause an irreversible change in the structure of DNA in a cell or cells which then has the potential to grow and produce a tumor. In addition, these same compounds cause other, as yet unidentified changes in the initiated cell and/or surrounding cells which allow the cells to divide in an uncontrolled manner.

For certain epigenetic carcinogens, it appears there may be a threshold dose; with others the biological effects leading to an increase in tumors are, under certain conditions of exposure, reversible. Although there are techniques that can be used to differentiate between genetic and epigenetic carcinogens, these techniques are not well enough developed at this time to provide unequivocal answers relative to the mechanisms by which a compound may be causing an increase in tumor incidence in experimental animals. The exception is that sufficiently well validated in vivo and in vitro techniques are available at this time to determine, with reasonable certainty, whether a compound is causing an increase in rat liver tumors by a genetic or epigenetic mechanism. In vivo and in vitro techniques for differentiating between genetic and epigenetic mechanisms for cancer induction in organs of species other than the liver of the rat have not yet been developed. When these techniques have been developed and appropriately validated, it may also be possible to determine with reasonable certainty whether a compound acts by a genetic or an epigenetic mechanism. As noted previously, the effects of epigenetic carcinogens may be, under certain conditions, reversible and there is evidence for thresholds for certain of these compounds. Therefore, with the advent of reliable assays, it may be possible to regulate human exposure to those chemicals adequately identified as epigenetic carcinogens with greater certainty and therefore less conservatively than compounds shown to increase tumor incidence in experimental animals by a genetic mechanism.

E. Structure-Activity Relationship

An estimate of the potential of a chemical to produce cancer in experimental animals and, by implication, in man can be obtained by comparing its structure with that of known carcinogenic chemicals. Of the various classes of compounds, those of particular concern are chemically reactive substances which act as direct alkylating or arylating agents, polyaromatic hydrocarbons, aromatic amines, aromatic nitro compounds, nitrosamines, and substituted hydrazines. However, subtle changes in the structures of various members of these and other classes of compounds markedly alter their carcinogenicity in experimental animals relative to other members of the class. In most instances the reasons for the marked differences in carcinogenicity related to small changes in structure are poorly understood. Thus, structure-activity considerations have a very limited usefulness in determining the potential carcinogenicity of chemicals to experimental animals and humans. With a better understanding of the reasons for these changes in biological activity related to changes in structure, this approach will become increasingly valuable.

F. Weight-of-Evidence

In evaluating the potential of a chemical to cause cancer in humans, it is important that all the data available on the chemical be considered. This is often referred to as the weight-of-evidence approach. An example of this approach is that recently proposed by Squire [17]. His scheme takes into account the various data elements available to evaluate the potential carcinogenic risk to man.

In support of the weight-of-evidence approach, the Committee on the Institutional Means for Assessment of Risks to Public Health of the National Academy of Sciences has recently stated [18] that "Every risk assessment involves consideration of case-specific factors, such as the quality of the data or the overall strength of the evidence."

III. RISK ASSESSMENT

Risk assessment is a multifaceted process involving components of hazard identification, hazard evaluation, risk evaluation, and risk or regulatory response. These features of risk assessment have been discussed by other authors [19]. Toxicology and epidemiology studies are fundamental to the hazard and risk evaluation process. Rates of adverse responses and variation of response may be determined by these procedures, usually under conditions where chemical dosages or exposure amounts greatly exceed the amounts expected under actual conditions of exposure for the chemical in question. Prediction of adverse chemical effects at low dosages or small exposures from data collected in animals or humans at high dosages is a complex problem because, among other things, there may often not be a linear proportionality between dose and response over the entire range from no exposure to high exposure. In fact, there is a considerable body of evidence for many chemicals that the response rates at low and high dosages are distinctly nonlinear. This feature probably applies to all forms of chronic toxicity, including cancer.

Theories of chemical carcinogenesis often emphasize that there must be a specific interaction of a carcinogen with genetic material and the insertion and fixation of a permanent change in the genome of cells of the target organ or tissue. These genetic changes may lead to uncontrolled cell growth and cancer and are thought to be linearly related to the amount of chemical reaching the DNA [20]. From these theories it follows that the expression of dose responsible for the carcinogenic response must be the amount of "active chemical" reaching the target DNA in a way that elicits the measured response. If no "active chemical" were to reach the target site then no response would be expected. On the other hand, if the "active chemical" reached the target site, then the frequency of response among a population of animals or humans would be a function of each individual's sensitivity (probability of showing an effect).

The state of the art in risk evaluation using animal bioassays or human epidemiological observations is primative and uncertain. Many procedures have been put forward, largely by statisticians and mathematicians, to predict the probability of response in populations exposed to specific chemicals at amounts equal to, and much less than, the amounts observed to cause effects in animals and humans. Recall here that there is almost always considerable uncertainty associated with epidemiologic observations in relation to the time of exposure, level of exposure, the duration of exposure, or the presence of confounding factors, such as individual lifestyles. Also there is qualitative and quantitative variability among the responses of different species that makes the extrapolation of the results in one species to another species an uncertain process. Nevertheless, since most of the known human carcinogens are also animal carcinogens, this uncertainty is not a major problem for qualitative extrapolation. Instead the issue of estimating risk quantitatively by extrapolating from the experimental range of dosages to the range of expected human exposures is of concern. One simple procedure is to identify a no-observed-effect-level for the chemical in animals or humans. A "safety factor" of 10–1000 or more may then be applied to the no-observed-effect-level to account for uncertainty of response within and between species or for population thresholds. This procedure is intuitively attractive, it tends to protect against adverse chemical effects, but it is not based on scientific considerations.

A. Low-Dosage Extrapolation Methodology

Many approaches to the problem of low-dose extrapolation and risk assessment have been devised. Linear extrapolation considers that the probability of tumor formation is directly proportional to carcinogen dose. Every dose, no matter how small, would be expected to carry some probability of tumor risk. An extension of this is linear interpolation between the lowest non-zero experimental dosage and the control [21]. The nonlinearity of most biological processes, including the absorption, metabolism, and excretion of chemicals, makes linear extrapolation or interpolation methodologies rather unappealing. Other statistical or stochastic models have been suggested to obviate the inherent problems of linear extrapolation. Among these are the probit, logit, and Weibull distributions, as well as the gamma multihit and multistage models [22]. These models also fail in one way or another to account for the mechanism of a chemical's toxic effect which may differ at high and low dosages and, therefore, do not seem to be biologically plausible. At best they only approximate the expected response at low dosages. Moreover, from observations in a given chronic animal bioassay, the various models may give very different low-dose risk estimates, and there is often inadequate biological evidence to decide upon the model of choice. One approach, which mixes science and policy, is to select the model that gives the most conservative estimate of risk even though this approach may not be supportable on scientific grounds. The choice of model therefore incorporates an additional uncertainty factor that should be reflected in the uncertainty of the risk estimate [23].

One risk assessment model employed by many regulatory agencies is the "linearized" multistage model [24] which replaces the linear term with a measure of the biological variability observed in tumor frequencies. This model predicts dose responses that are approximately linear at low doses and, thus, in most cases leads to no appreciable difference in risk estimates between the linear model and the linearized multistage model.

More recently models have been advanced which utilize pharmacokinetic information to predict the concentration of "active chemical" at relevant reactive sites. In comparison to models typically used for low-dose extrapolation, these models account for nonlinear kinetics and show that failure to include nonlinear terms may lead to the overestimation of risk by several orders of magnitude [25–28]. Additional efforts have been made to expand the multistage model to include a consideration of time to tumor [29]. Indeed, such approaches provide additional information, although many bioassays fail to collect the data necessary to include time to tumor in the analysis of risk.

The importance of information concerning the latent period for tumor induction is emphasized clearly by a recent report that the relationship between dose and latent period may not be linear [13]. Nitrosodiethylamine, a potent hepatocarcinogen, was administered to Old World monkeys at varying dosages. Dosages of 10.0, 20.0, and 40.0 mg/kg body weight each induced tumors, and the latent period required for tumor induction was inversely related to dose in a linear fashion. At dosages of 1.0 and 5.0 mg/kg body weight, however, the tumor latency expected from this linear relationship was not found. In fact the monkeys given 1.0 mg/kg body weight would have been predicted to have developed tumors at 60 months, although the group was tumor-free after 80 months of observation. In primates, therefore, linear relationship between dose and tumor latency cannot be assumed.

B. Risk Evaluation for Formaldehyde Toxicity

A chronic toxicity and oncogenicity study of inhaled formaldehyde in rats and mice demonstrated that formaldehyde was carcinogenic for both species. Rats were more sensitive than mice, however, and 50% of rats exposed to the highest exposure concentration of 14.3 ppm formaldehyde (6 hr/day, 5 days/week) for up to 24 months had squamous cell carcinomas in the nasal passages. Approximately 1% of the mice exposed to this concentration under identical conditions developed nasal tumors. Formaldehyde in the air at 5.6 ppm induced fewer nasal tumors; approximately a 1% incidence in the rat and none in mice. There were no squamous cell carcinomas in the nasal passages of either rats or mice exposed to 2 ppm of formaldehyde or in controls. Benign polyploid adenomas were observed in the nasal passages of some treated and control rats but these lesions were not statistically significant [30]. Clearly, formaldehyde is an animal carcinogen, although it is of interest that one species is far more sensitive than another. Quantitatively, therefore, rats do not predict the incidence of tumors to be expected in mice and vice versa. The species response, and differences, may be relevant to human risk assessment, but since carcinogenicity in humans has not been associated with formaldehyde exposure, the appropriate predictive animal model is unknown [31].

One recent quantitative risk assessment on formaldehyde was conducted by a regulatory agency, the Consumer Product Safety Commission (CPSC), by fitting the multistage quantal response model to the incidence of squamous cell carcinomas in rats [32]. In this analysis, humans were assumed to be equally as sensitive as rats to the carcinogenicity of formaldehyde and that formaldehyde acted on genetic material in the same concentration-time product relationship for both species to elicit similar responses. The product of the concentration of formaldehyde in ambient air and the duration of exposure was taken as the measure of formaldehyde dose at the target site.

As explained above, risk estimates based solely on response versus administered dose may be erroneous if nonlinear kinetics are involved in the delivery of the "active chemical" to the target site [33]. Since the dose response for formaldehyde-induced squamous cell carcinoma in the nasal passages of rats is distinctly nonlinear, it follows that there may be a number of protective barriers and/or detoxification mechanisms that limit the amount of formaldehyde reaching target cells [30]. For example, the mucous blanket and mucociliary clearance apparatus which protect the nasal epithelium under normal conditions may limit the amount of formaldehyde delivered to target cells at low concentrations as contrasted with high concentrations. In fact, formaldehyde causes mucostasis and ciliastasia in the nasal passages of rats at 6 ppm and above. Effects at 2 ppm are slight and there is no effect at 0.5 ppm [31]. Moreover, at high concentrations of formaldehyde (6 or 15 ppm) cell death and cell proliferation are enhanced [31] which may allow exogenous formaldehyde direct access to the DNA of proliferating cells in the absence of full protection by the mucous blanket. Under these conditions, the likelihood of genotoxic events may be increased which might explain the distinct nonlinearity of the formaldehyde-induced carcinogenic response in rodents. A variety of studies have also demonstrated that rats and mice exposed to the same ambient air concentration of formaldehyde do not receive the same dose on the nasal epithelium. In fact, mice receive a dose to the nasal epithelium one-half the size of that delivered to the nasal epithelium of the rat at 15 ppm. This is accounted for by the differential response in intensity of the respiratory depression reflex in rats and mice elicited by sensory irritants.

In rodents, formaldehyde toxicity and carcinogenicity are limited to the upper respiratory tract indicating that formaldehyde in an "active" form is not delivered to distant sites to cause adverse effects. Presumably a similar situation would apply in humans. Recent studies have shown that the concentration of formaldehyde in the blood of rats and humans is not elevated following exposure to airborne formaldehyde [33]. Moreover, formaldehyde is a normal endogenous biochemical and an active metabolic capability exists for the normal metabolism of formaldehyde. It is unlikely, therefore, that exposure to low concentrations of formaldehyde results in formaldehydes reaching distant target sites or actual target sites in a linear fashion. Indeed, it appears likely that a series of nonlinear functions may serve to limit formaldehyde access to DNA, the presumed target site. From the above discussion, it is evident that for formaldehyde risk evaluation the independent variable, dose, in a quantitative risk extrapolation should reflect the concentration of the "active chemical" at the target site rather than the amount of the parent compound in ambient air. The effect of using delivered dose instead of administered dose in risk assessments of formaldehyde has been considered and risk estimates are much less conservative in the former [34]. The utilization of mechanistic information in quantitative risk assessment may provide a stronger scientific basis for extrapolation to human risk than otherwise would be possible.

C. Inorganic Arsenic Carcinogenicity

Although numerous animal studies have failed to detect carcinogenicity for inorganic arsenic, there is clear evidence in humans that arsenic may induce respiratory tract and skin cancer [35]. In order to establish safe exposure limits, a regulatory agency has conducted a quantitative risk assessment to develop a final inorganic arsenic standard. These analyses have been made from the results of epidemiological studies conducted in copper smelter workers. The epidemiological data confirmed a dose-response relationship for arsenic exposure and lung cancer risk. In fact, these studies led to the estimation of an excess risk of lung cancer from arsenic exposure at levels less than the permissible exposure limit previously established by the Occupational Safety and Health Administration (OSHA; 500 $\mu g/m^3$). These epidemiology studies measured actual risks at high arsenic exposure and are to be contrasted with the risks predicted from low-dosage extrapolation models at low arsenic exposure. Utilizing a linear model for low-dosage extrapolation, OSHA concluded that for inorganic arsenic exposure the risk for a 45-year working lifetime leads to an excess risk of 8 deaths per 1000 at 10 $\mu g/m^3$, 40 deaths per 1000 at 50 $\mu g/m^3$ and 400 deaths per 1000 at 500 $\mu g/m^3$. These conclusions assume that there is no threshold for carcinogenicity of inorganic arsenic. Additional details of the mechanism of carcinogenicity for inorganic arsenic, therefore, are not considered by this model and biological plausibility for the model has not been shown.

Additional analysis of the inorganic arsenic epidemiological data has led to the suggestion that arsenic carcinogenicity may be understood in terms of a multistage mechanism [36]. Evidence has been cited that arsenic acts at a late stage in the carcinogenic process and that there is an increasing excess of lung cancer mortality risk with increasing age at initial exposure. While this conclusion is speculative, since no experimental evidence exists that arsenic has a role in a multistage cellular transformation process, it demonstrates that analysis of patterns of excess risk depending on exposure duration, age at initial exposure, and time since termination of exposure may be useful in identifying stages within a carcinogenic transformation process that are affected by exposure. Further pursuit of such a hypothesis might be highly useful in providing more predictive and meaningful risk assessment and/or evaluation procedures.

One conclusion from the analysis of the arsenic data is important to industrial epidemiologists. That is, that a complete work history is necessary in order to determine any exposure before and subsequent to the particular employment being studied. Industry should attempt to maintain adequate records of work histories throughout each employee's career.

IV. CONCLUSION

Toxicology and epidemiology studies play an important role in hazard identification, hazard evaluation, risk evaluation, and risk regulation. However, it is important that all data be evaluated in accordance with the limits imposed by science. In this regard, as noted previously, the inclusion of mechanistic information is most valuable. Further work to delineate mechanisms of toxicity and carcinogenicity must therefore be a part of the scientific process of hazard and risk evaluation.

REFERENCES

1. L. Tomatis, Long-term and short-term screening assays for carcinogens: A critical appraisal, *IARC Monographs Supplement 2*, IARC, Lyon, France, 1980.
2. Percivall Pott, *Chirurgical Observations Relative to the Cataract, the Polypus of the Nose, the Cancer of the Scrotum, the Different Kinds of Ruptures, and the Mortification of the Toes and Feet*, Hawes, Clarke and Collins, London (1775).
3. J. L. Creech, Jr., and M. N. Johnson, Angiosarcoma of the liver in the manufacture of polyvinyl chloride, *J. Occup. Med., 16*:150 (1974).
4. Chemicals and industrial processes associated with cancer in humans, *IARC Monographs Supplement 1*, IARC, Lyon, France, 1979.
5. J. Cairns, The origin of human cancers, *Nature*, 289:353 (1981).
6. Evaluation of the carcinogenic risk of chemicals to humans: Some food additives, feed additives and naturally occurring substances, *IARC Monograph, 31*:19, IARC, Lyon, France, 1983.
7. A. W. Andrews, L. H. Thibault, and W. Lijinski, The relationship between mutagenicity and carcinogenicity of some nitrosamines, *Mutat. Res., 51*:311 (1978).
8. A. W. Andrews, L. H. Thibault, and W. Lijinski. The relationship between mutagenicity and carcinogenicity of some nitrosamines, *Mutat. Res., 51*:319 (1978).
9. H. Bartsch, C. Malaveille, A. M. Camus, G. Martel-Planche, G. Brun, A. Hautefeuille, N. Sabadie, A. Barbin, T. Kuroki, C. Drevon, C. Picolli, and R. Montesano, Bacterial and mammalian mutagenicity tests: Validation and comparative studies on 180 chemicals, in *Molecular and Cellular Aspects of Carcinogen Screening Tests*, (R. Montesano, H. Bartsch and L. Tomatis, eds.), IARC Scientific Publications 27:179, IARC, Lyon, France, 1980.
10. M. M. Coombs, C. Dixon, and A. M. Kissonerghis, Evaluation of the mutagenicity of compounds of known carcinogenicity, belonging to the benz(a)anthracene, chrysene and cyclopenta(a)phenanthrene series, using Ames's test, *Cancer Res., 36*:4524 (1976).

11. H. R. Glatt, H. Schwind, F. Zajdela, A. Croisy, P. C. Jacquignon, and F. Oesch, Mutagenicity of 43 structurally related heterocyclic compounds and its relationship to their carcinogenicity, *Mutat. Res., 66*:307 (1979).

12. I. F. H. Purchase, Inter-species comparison of carcinogenicity, *Br. J. Cancer, 41*:454 (1980).

13. R. H. Adamson and S. M. Sieber, Chemical carcinogenesis studies in non-human primates, in *Organ and Species Specificity in Chemical Carcinogenesis*, (R. Langenbach, S. Nesnow and J. M. Rice, eds.), Plenum Publishing Corporation, New York, 1983.

14. Some monomers, plastics and synthetic elastomers, and acrolein, *IARC Monograph 19*, IARC, Lyon, France, 1979.

15. *OECD Guidelines for Testing Chemicals*, Organisation for Economic Cooperation and Development, OECD Publications Center, Washington, DC, 1981.

16. Proposed Guidelines for Registering Pesticides in the U.S.: Hazard evaluation; humans and domestic animals, *Fed. Reg., 43*:37336, (1978).

17. R. A. Squire, Ranking animal carcinogens: A proposed regulatory approach, *Science, 214*:877 (1981).

18. *Risk Assessment in the Federal Government: Managing the Process.* National Research Council, Committee on the Institutional Means for Assessment of Risks to Public Health, National Academy Press, 1983.

19. P. F. Deisler, Jr., A goal-oriented approach to reducing industrially related carcinogenic risks, *Drug Metab. Rev., 13*:875 (1982).

20. P. Armitage and R. Doll, The age distribution of cancer and a multistage theory of carcinogenesis, *Br. J. Cancer, 8*:1 (1954).

21. D. W. Gaylor and R. L. Kodell, Linear interpolation algorithm for low dose risk assessment of toxic substances, *J. Environ. Pathol. Toxicol., 4*:305 (1980).

22. D. R. Krewski and J. Van Ryzin, Dose response models for quantal response toxicity data, in *Statistics and Related Topics*, (M. Csorgo, D. Dawson, J. N. K. Rao and E. Saleh, eds.), North Holland Publishing Company, Amsterdam, 1981.

23. S. Wong, Low dose extrapolation: Inference and design under the multistage model. Presented before the American Statistical Association, August, 1983.

24. K. S. Crump and W. W. Watson, A Fortran program to extrapolate dichotomous animal carcinogenicity data to low doses, Department of Mathematics and Statistics, Louisiana Tech University (1979).

25. D. G. Hoel, N. L. Kaplan, and M. W. Anderson, Implications of nonlinear kinetics on risk estimation in carcinogenesis, *Science, 219*:1032 (1983).

26. J. Cornfield, Carcinogenic risk assessment, *Science,* 198:693 (1977).
27. P. J. Gehring and G. E. Blau, Mechanisms of carcinogenesis: Dose response, *J. Environ. Pathol. Toxicol., 1*:163 (1977).
28. M. W. Anderson, D. G. Hoel, and N. L., Kaplan, A general scheme for the incorporation of pharmacokinetics in low-dose risk estimation for chemical carcinogenesis: Example—vinyl chloride, *Toxicol. Appl. Pharmacol., 55*:154 (1980).
29. H. O. Hartley and R. L. Sielken, Jr., Estimation of "safe doses" in carcinogenic experiments, *Biometrics, 33*:1 (1977).
30. W. D. Kerns, K. L. Pavkov, D. J. Donofrio, E. J. Gralla, and J. A. Swenberg, Carcinogenicity of formaldehyde in rats and mice after long-term inhalation exposure, *Cancer Res., 43*:4382 (1983).
31. J. A. Swenberg, C. S. Barrow, C. J. Boreiko, H. d'A. Heck, R. J. Levine, K. T. Morgan, and T. B. Starr, Non-linear biological responses to formaldehyde and their implications for carcinogenic risk assessment, *Carcinogenesis, 4*:945 (1983).
32. Consumer Product Safety Commission, Part IV: Consumer Product Safety Commission ban of urea formaldehyde foam insulation, withdrawal of proposed labeling rule, and denial of petition to issue a standard, *Fed. Reg., 47*:14366 (1982).
33. H. d'A. Heck, M. Casanova-Schmitz, P. B. Dodd, E. N. Schachter, T. Witek, and T. Tosun, Formaldehyde (FA) concentrations in the blood of humans and F-344 rats exposed to FA under controlled conditions, *Toxicologist,* in press (1984).
34. T. B. Starr, Mechanisms of formaldehyde toxicity and risk evaluation, in *Formaldehyde: Toxicology, Epidemiology, and Mechanisms,* (J. J. Clary, J. E. Gibson and R. S. Waritz, eds.), Marcel Dekker, Inc., New York, in press, 1983.
35. Department of Labor, Occupational Safety and Health Administration, Occupation exposure to inorganic arsenic, *Fed. Reg., 48*:1864 (1983).
36. C. C. Brown and K. C. Chu, Implications of the multistage theory of carcinogenesis applied to occupational arsenic exposure, *J. Nat. Cancer Inst., 70*:455 (1983).

4

FEDERAL RESEARCH AIMED AT REDUCING CANCER RISKS

Michael Gough
Office of Technology Assessment
Congress of the United States
Washington, D.C.

I. INTRODUCTION

Federal cancer research runs the gamut from basic biological research through discrete, focused risk assessments in support of regulations, to new approaches in treatment and palliation of cancer
patients. The federal government spends at a rate of over a billion
dollars a year on cancer (see Table 1), and it supports scientific inquiries in universities, hospitals, profit and nonprofit private laboratories, and government facilities.

Federally supported research activities can be categorized in
several ways. For instance, reasonable divisions can be drawn along
the lines of disciplines or of the locations of the research efforts.
In this chapter, the activities will be divided, according to objectives, into five groups: (1) *basic research* directed at understanding
the biology of cancer, (2) *identification* of substances, exposures,
and behaviors that are cancer hazards *and estimation of risks* they
pose, (3) development of *methods to control and reduce risks*, (4)
inquiries into possible *prophylaxis against risks*, and (5) research
into and dissemination of advances in *medical care*. This chapter is
focused on items (1) and (4) with some attention to (2) and little
mention of the others.

Support of basic research which, when contemplated and plan-
ned, is often far away from any "payoff" is seen by most people
as an appropriate function of the federal government. In fact, as
will be described, much of our expanding information about cancer biology depends on basic research in other subdisciplines of
biology. The great majority of such research was and is supported
by the federal government, the National Science Foundation
(NSF) and the National Institutes of Health (NIH).

Identification of cancer risks through testing of substances using
animals is not limited to federal activities but is also carried out by

Table 1 Federal Funding of Cancer-Related Activities by the Federal Government, 1982

Organizations	$ (Thousands)
National Cancer Institute	943,029
Other institutes of the National Institutes of Health	135,747
Other components of the Department of Health and Human Services (excluding NIH)	11,296
Consumer Product Safety Commission	2,500
Department of Agriculture	79,000
Department of Labor, Occupational Safety and Health Administration	800
Environmental Protection Agency	16,661
National Science Foundation	6,000
Nuclear Regulatory Commission	1,600
Veterans Administration	11,500
Total	1,216,677

Source: NCI [1]

industrial firms and trade associations. This chapter will discuss some activities of the National Toxicology Program (NTP) and the National Center of Toxicological Research (NCTR) in test development, standardization, execution, and interpretation. Federal records systems that are useful in epidemiologic studies of the occurrence of human cancers are described here (see also Chapters 1 and 7).

Federal efforts to control and reduce carcinogenic risks result in the publication of information documents, suggestions for control methods, and regulations to force the installation of controls. Both the Environmental Protection Agency (EPA) and the National Institute for Occupational Safety and Health (NIOSH) produce documents that describe the agencies' assessment of the level of risk from various substances. These documents have no regulatory force, but they play the important function of influencing decisions to control and to reduce exposures. NIOSH, through its Division of Control Technologies, has organized workshops to bring together experts from the private and public sectors to discuss the best methods to control health risks. These activities go beyond providing information about hazards to providing information about controls. Finally, the Occupational Safety and Health Administration (OSHA) issues regulations that direct employers to reduce exposures to specified levels (see Chapter 9). These efforts at providing information and incentives to control exposures, although dependent on research, are not discussed in this chapter. A general discussion of workplace safety and health is available in *Controls for Health and Safety in the Workplace* [2].

The importance of dietary factors in cancer causation has long been recognized (see Chapter 1), but the idea that some foods contain "anticarcinogens" has become especially important in the 1980's [3–5]. Investigations of the possibility that some substances offer *prophylaxis against the effects of carcinogens* are now underway, and they are described in this chapter.

The federal government, through the National Cancer Institute (NCI) is the leader in efforts to treat cancer. Although much of that activity is research, it is not directed at preventing cancer, and will not be discussed here. The interested reader is referred to the annual *National Cancer Program: Director's Report and Annual Plan*, which is available from the Office of Cancer Communications, National Cancer Institute, Bethesda, MD 20205.

II. BASIC RESEARCH

In 1953, James Watson, a biologist, and Frances Crick, a physicist, published a short paper in *Nature* that described the structure of the genetic material, DNA [6]. Watson's book *The Double Helix* [8], which describes the discovery of the structure of DNA, opens with the sentence, "I have never seen Francis Crick in a modest mood."* Evidently, neither Watson nor Crick was feeling humble when writing a closing sentence of their paper:

---

*Crick has not written a book about the discovery, but he said he had thought of a title for such a book. He would call it *The Loose Screw*. His first sentence would be, "Jim [Watson] was always clumsy with his hands. One had only to see him peel an orange . . . " [7].

It has not escaped our notice that the specific pairing we have postulated immediately suggests a possible copying mechanism for the genetic material.

The elegance of the now familiar double helix structure immediately convinced most scientists that Watson and Crick were correct. The structure of DNA and its method of replication to guarantee that genetic information was passed correctly from cell to daughter cell and from generation to generation was known. It was a watershed in the history of science.

Was this exciting discovery to remain limited to the purview of molecular biologists? For awhile, yes. Until the advent of "genetic engineering" in the 1970s, studying the discrete bits of DNA involved in making the biology of a cancer cell different from a normal cell was impossible.

A. The Beginning of Genetic Engineering

Hamilton O. Smith's Nobel lecture [9] describes the discovery of "restriction enzymes" that cut DNA molecules at specific points, which opened the way to the isolation and identification of particular pieces of DNA, such as "cancer genes." The ability to cut DNA molecules at specific sites and to recombine pieces of DNA from different organs and organisms made possible the discovery of the restriction enzymes and provided biologists with an unprecedented opportunity to study DNA and gene function.

In 1968, Smith, at Johns Hopkins University and supported by a NSF grant, was studying the transfer of genetic information from one bacterium to another. He used a technique that involved extracting DNA from the "donor" bacterium and mixing the "naked DNA" with a "recipient" cell.* For technical reasons, Smith included DNA from an unrelated bacterial virus in his experiment, and he was surprised that the viral DNA was degraded

---

*This same technique had been used more than two decades earlier to show that DNA is the genetic material [10]. Until then, based on theoretical grounds, many scientists had thought that the genetic material must be protein.

during its interaction with the recipient cell, while the bacterial DNA was not. In other words, the recipient cells degraded unrelated or "foreign" DNA, but did not degrade DNA from the same cell type or "self" DNA.

Smith was steeped in the lore of an exotic branch of microbial genetics that flourished in the 1950s and 1960s. A number of biologists, beginning with S. Luria (Nobel Prize, 1969, for research in another area of genetics) and supported almost exclusively by federal funds, had studied "restriction" of the growth of bacterial viruses. Simply put, they observed that viruses previously grown on one strain of bacteria would grow with only very low efficiency on related but not identical strains [11,12].

Shortly before making his observation that the foreign DNA was degraded, Smith had read a paper that said that "restriction" involved degradation of DNA. In a series of brilliant experiments, Smith and his colleagues showed that a single bacterial enzyme was responsible for the degradation and that the enzyme always cut the DNA at the same sequence of nucleotides [13]. Every DNA fragment produced by the enzyme had identical ends. From these, it became a relatively simple exercise to rejoin the fragments. And, the fragments could be rejoined in different sequences. Even more importantly, fragments of DNA from different organisms could be rejoined. Genetic engineering was born.

Soon after making his initial observations, Smith (personal communication, 1983) wrote about the properties of the restriction enzyme to Daniel Nathans, a colleague at Hopkins who was on sabbatical in Israel. Nathans seized upon the availability of the new tool and immediately applied it to cutting up and analyzing the DNA of simian virus 40 (SV 40). This virus is a monkey tumor virus that was discovered as a contaminant of the cell cultures used to prepare Salk polio vaccine. Simian virus 40 is easily grown in the laboratory and was an early, favorite subject of study by tumor virologists. Using the techniques made possible by Smith's work, Nathans was able to show which parts of the viral DNA coded for various proteins that were involved in the virus' converting a normal cell into a cancer cell. (Nathans and W. Arber, a Swiss scientist who had studied restriction, shared the 1978 Nobel Prize with Smith.)

The discovery and isolation of scores of restriction enzymes quickly followed. The flexibility gained from having different enzymes that cut DNA at different locations, which allowed the isolation of many different fragments from the same DNA, has fueled the rapid growth of biotechnology [13,14]. The burgeoning biotechnology industry is one result of the federal government's support of basic biologic research. Another is the very rapid progress in our understanding of the biology of cancer.

B. Recombinant DNA Techniques in the Understanding of Cancer

1. The Identification of the First Human Cancer Virus

Knowing what the DNA of a virus "looks like' through recombinant DNA techniques allows scientists to search for viral DNA inside tumor cells. During 1981, scientists at the NCI successfully isolated and characterized a virus that causes a rare human leukemia.

Since its initial discovery, the human cancer virus (HTLV for human T-cell leukemia virus) has been reported throughout the world, but in all cases in small geographical regions. Although the virus causes cancer, it is not infectious in the sense that influenza viruses are, and the method of its spread is not yet understood. Furthermore, in those areas where HTLV is found, it is commonly detectable in persons who do not have leukemia. The conditions following infection that are necessary for the development of cancer remain to be understood. Human T-cell leukemia virus itself was a candidate for an etiologic agent in acquired immunity deficiency syndrome (AIDS) because it attacks the same cells rendered defective in AIDS [15]. Early in 1984, Robert Gallo and colleagues at NIH and scientists in France showed that a virus closely related to HTLV is associated with AIDS.

The percentage of human cancer caused by viruses is thought to be small [3,4], but the successes achieved in preparing vaccines against other viral diseases makes the discovery of HTLV and other viruses associated with human cancers [1] especially important. It may be that vaccines can be developed against viral-caused or -associated cancer.

2. The Role of Genetic Changes in Cancer

For years most scientists have accepted the idea that cancer involves DNA. Perhaps the most simple imaginable model to test that hypothesis is to look at the DNA of a tumor cell to see if it is, in fact, different from a normal cell. A number of laboratories have used a variety of clever tricks developed in the study of the genetics of bacterial viruses and recombinant DNA techniques to look at tumor cell DNA.

R. Weinberg's laboratory at MIT and M. Wigler's at Cold Spring Harbor Laboratory isolated "cancer genes" from human bladder tumors and using genetic engineering techniques "grew" them. The human cancer gene, called *ras* for reasons that need not concern us here, was shown to resemble closely both a viral oncogene (a gene that is carried by cancer viruses that is involved in cancer), and a gene found in normal human cells. What was more surprising was that the viral oncogene differed from the normal human gene at exactly the same nucleotide as the bladder tumor gene. Therefore, these studies showed that genes from three different biological sources were closely related. *A single nucleotide change distinguishes a "normal" gene from a "cancer" gene.* And a change at the same location distinguishes both those genes from an oncogene in a cancer virus. Subsequently, it has been found that other single nucleotide changes at different locations in the DNA are sufficient to shift the "normal" gene to a cancer gene. Weinberg has written a popularized account in the *Atlantic Monthly* [16] and a more technical article in *Scientific American* [17].

A critical point in these experiments was an assay for the cancer gene. The assay showed that DNA from cancer cells "transformed" other cells in culture to behave like tumor cells. The transformed cells grow differently from nontransformed cells, and they cause tumors when injected into healthy animals. Nontransformed cells do not.

But, wait, said many scientists. The assay used by Weigle and Weinstein involves the use of special kind of cell as a recipient of the DNA. The special cells are called NIH 3T3 cells, or 3T3, for short. Most attempts to grow mammalian cells in culture fail; the cells die after going through a few divisions. In the successful cases, such as 3T3, the cells go through a "crisis," and the survivors are immortal and capable of continual growth in culture medium. Tumor cells are also immortal, and the argument was made that although the bladder tumor DNA work was interesting, it might not mean much because 3T3 cells were already on the road to behaving like tumor cells. The argument was bolstered by the fact that the bladder tumor DNA could not transform normal cells (nonimmortal cells) into tumor like cells.

Since 3T3 cells can be viewed as having moved part of the way along the path to transformation, it can be suggested that the human bladder tumor gene was sufficient to push it the rest of the way. Also, this line of reasoning suggests that the bladder cancer gene is a "late" function; it converts already immortal cultured cells into transformed cells. Given the assumption that the transformed or tumorous state is a result of genetic changes, it is reasonable to suppose that introducing appropriate "early-acting" genes into a normal cell in combination with the "late-acting" gene from the human bladder tumor would be sufficient for transformation.

In fact, this was found to be the case. Equally fascinating, the early function can be supplied by genes from different viruses. Therefore, the interaction between early and late functions is not restricted to a gene from a particular virus being necessary to interact with the human bladder gene. Furthermore, late genes can interact with early genes from other sources to transform normal cells [18,19]. These interactions are consistent with the idea that early genes from whatever sources are similar to each other, that late genes share similarities, and that there may be a limited number of both. If there were many early and late genes with strict requirements for interactions, it would not favor a successful interaction between a human bladder late-acting gene and early genes from different sources.

3. Steps Along the Way to Cancer

There is a great deal of speculation and some evidence for the early event in carcinogenesis involving a rearrangement in the structure of DNA [20]. As we have already seen, the late event seems to be more simple and can involve an alteration of a single nucleotide.

In tissue culture cells, an early step along the way to transformation is the cell's becoming immortal; that is, capable of unlimited cell divisions. If an analogous step occurs in the cells of an animal, it could result in a body cell growing and dividing at a rate greater than normal. The extra growth, in turn, might facilitate the occurrence of mutations. When a mutation analogous to that seen in the human bladder tumor occurs, the cell would be converted into a tumor cell. The beauty of such models is that they generate ideas, and the available laboratory methods allow the testing of those ideas.

4. A Demonstrated Relationship Between Chemical Carcinogenesis and Cancer Genes

Initiation of cancer is thought to involve an interaction with DNA. The interactions with DNA that most concern us right now are those from chemicals in the environment. Knowing the results of the studies that showed that a gene from human bladder cancers can cause the transformation of "immortal" cells suggests an experiment to see if chemicals can cause cells to become immortal. In other words, can a chemical (or physical) insult substitute for the early function that was introduced by viral genes in the experiments discussed above.

Newbold and Overell [21] treated hamster cells with a chemical mutagen or x-rays (a physical mutagen) and isolated cells that were made immortal as a result of the exposure. The mutagenized cells were transformable by the human bladder cancer gene. This experiment shows that a mutagen is sufficient to cause the early event(s) along the road to transformation. It provides a direct link between chemicals and cancer causation.

The ability to dissect the transformation events into an immortalization event and a later event will likely be of great importance to toxicologists in their studies of carcinogenesis. The resultant sharpening of toxicology's tools may be one of the earliest payoffs from the recent rapid progress in understanding the molecular biology of the cancer cell.

5. The Relationship Between a Human Protein of Known Function and a Protein Associated With Cancer Causation

One of the frustrating things about the human bladder tumor genes is that little is known about the proteins produced by their "normal" analogs. However, basic research in another area of biology has shown that a human protein known to be involved in wound healing is closely related to a protein known to be important in cancer.

In May 1983, a partial amino acid sequence of the protein (platelet-derived growth factor) was published in *Science* [22]. R. Doolittle, as part of his ongoing research into evolution, copied the amino acid sequence into a computer. He discovered that 61 of the 70 known amino acids matched the amino acids present in a protein made by a monkey cancer virus. A paper published in July 1983 [23] explores the relationship of the two proteins.

It is quite a simple matter to draw a picture of how the activities of the two proteins can be related. The human protein is known to promote healing by stimulating cell multiplication. The monkey cancer virus gene, by influencing cell multiplication, could be associated with cancer by causing a step analogous to the immortalization required to transform cells in culture.

C. The General Nature of "Cancer Genes"

All of the experiments that show the role of altered genes in cancer causation and transformation depend to some extent on the oncogenes carried by cancer viruses. It is incorrect to conclude that the viral location of those genes is of great importance. Instead, the cancer genes, whether found in a virus or in an animal cell, are of animal origin. Those found in viruses were picked up from animal cells by the virus, but they are merely along for the ride. The cancer viruses that are so useful in studying cancer are lucky happenstances because they provide a convenient mechanism to study cancer genes, but as a respected authority expresses it [24],

The viruses carrying oncogenes are uncommon. . . . There is no reason to believe, for the moment, that tumorigenesis by

[viruses] carrying oncogenes is a common . . . form of onco-
genesis. It is a wonderful gift of nature that these things exist.
But they arise very rarely. And I think, myself, that the virus
carrying an oncogene has no evolutionary significance. We know
that when we grow these viruses in the laboratory, the oncogene
is lost very easily. It's the experimentalist, not selection in
nature, that preserves the oncogene.

Therefore, the studies are looking at genes of animal or human
origin, and they provide information about the genetic changes involved in cancer. It is not immediately apparent where these research efforts will lead, but their application to understanding cancer is much more direct than the experiments with bacteria and
bacterial viruses of 20 and 30 years ago. And seeing what has been
reaped from those studies makes me, at least, expect rapid
progress and fairly early "practical" applications to preventing
cancer.

III. IDENTIFICATION OF CARCINOGENIC HAZARDS
AND ESTIMATION OF CANCER RISKS

A.   Development and Execution of Tests for
Carcinogenic Substances

1. The National Toxicology Program

The federal government's testing of substances for carcinogens is
centered in the National Toxicology Program (NTP). Headquar-
tered at the National Institute of Environmental Health Sciences,
the NTP conducts testing and test development in its own laboratories and sponsors grant and contract-supported research in other
federal laboratories, universities, and private laboratories. It publishes an annual plan and a quarterly *NTP Technical Bulletin*
which are available through Dr. Larry Hart, NTP, P.O. Box 12233,
Research Triangle Park, NC 27709. A description of the NTP's research and testing programs has recently been published [25].
    The *1983 Annual Plan* [26] lists 160 chemicals that were in the
chronic phase of bioassay for carcinogenicity, and 45 that were in
the prechronic phases. In 1982, NTP completed the peer review of

21 bioassays, and 26 are scheduled for completion in 1983. The NIOSH actively participates in the selection of substances to be tested by NTP. Reflecting the complex exposures typical of industry, NIOSH has sponsored tests of synthetic machine oils, pyrolysis effluents from foundry mold binders, interactions between ethanol or disulfiram and 1,2-dichloroethane, mixtures such as diesel exhaust and coal dusts, and individual substances such as ethylene oxide. The protocols and justifications for these studies are being peer reviewed, and adjustments in the experiments can be made in response to comments of peer reviewers.

In addition to executing tests, NTP has been active in modifying the protocol for the carcinogenic bioassay. The basic design of the bioassay was laid down in a 1976 publication [27], and its importance is illustrated by Table 2. It can be seen that two testing protocols proposed by the Environmental Protection Agency (EPA), one under the Toxic Substances Control Act and the other under the Federal Insecticide Fungicide and Rodenticide Act, closely followed the 1976 proposal. NTP has modified the protocol depending on the nature of the substance under test, and it has made some general changes such as increasing the number of doses from two to three. Other changes have also been incorporated and considered, and during 1983, NTP convened a blue-ribbon panel to reconsider the 1976 protocol. The panel, composed of scientists from a number of scientific disciplines and representing industry, government, labor, environmental groups, and universities, expects to complete a draft for public review in 1984.

In addition to bioassays, NTP is also very active in the development and execution of short-term tests [4]. Of particular importance to cancer, is the exploration of in vivo tests for organ-specific effects of carcinogenic substances. These tests, if validated, may become important in understanding the interactions between initiators, promoters, and cocarcinogens.

In the five years of its existence, the NTP has organized the federal government's "routine" testing of carcinogens into a smoothly working system. The results of the tests are not always greeted as accurate or important for human health, but those criticisms can be levelled at any test results which displease the critic.

Table 2 Guidelines for Bioassay in Small Rodents

	NCI[a]	FIFRA	TSCA
Endpoint	Carcinogenicity	Oncogenicity	Oncogenicity
Study plan			
Animal species	2, rats and mice	2, rats and mice	2, rats and mice
Number of animals at each dose	50 males, 50 females	50 males, 50 females	50 males, 50 females
Dosages	2, MTD, MTD/2, or MTD/4 plus no-dosage control	3, MTD, MTD/2, or MTD/4, MTD/4 or MTD/8 plus dose control	3, HDL, HDL/2, or HDL/4, HDL/4 or HDL/10 plus no-dosage control
Dosing regimen			
Start	At 6 weeks of age	In utero or at 6 weeks	At 6 weeks of age
End	At 24 months of age	Mice, 18–24 mos; rats, 24–30	At 24–30 months of age
Observation period	3–6 months after end of dosing	N.S.	N.S.

Organs and tissues to be examined	All animals; external and histo-pathologic examination (approx. 30 organs and tissues)	All animals; external examination; some animals; pathologic exam of 30 organs and tissues, other animals, fewer organs and tissues	All animals; external and histo-pathologic examination (approx. 30 organs and tissue)[b]
Personnel qualifications:			
Study director	N.S.	N.S.	Responsibilities detailed
Pathologist	Board-qualified	N.S.	Board-certified or equivalent
Animal husbandry	N.S.	N.S.	Board-certified vet. or equivalent
Cost estimate	N.S.	N.S.	$400,000 b 160,000

[a]The NCI Guidelines specify the indicated minimum requirements. They allow for flexibility in experimental design so long as the minimum requirements are met.
[b]EPA estimates that the 40,000 microscope slides produced in this examination will require more than 3/4 of a year of a pathologist's time for analysis.
Abbreviations: MTD, Maximum tolerated dose, causes minor acute toxicity; HDL, High-dose level, causes some acute toxicity; N.S., Not specified.
Source: Office of Technology Assessment [4]

Very much on the positive side, however, NTP has made serious efforts to bring scientists from all sectors of the economy into its planning and review activities. Furthermore, its recognizing that the "standard bioassay" no longer satisfies scientists who expect that noncostly modifications can improve the information produced from the tests, is an important step in keeping testing current with new knowledge.

2. National Center for Toxicological Research

The National Center for Toxicological Research (NCTR), part of the Food and Drug Administration, is located at Jefferson, Arkansas. The agency is described in *Research Activities Tracking System (RATS),* which is available from Dr. Ronald Hart, Director, NCTR, Jefferson, AK 72079.

NCTR participates in the NTP and conducts some tests for it. However, its director (personal communication, 1983) sees the NCTR as filling a unique role in the federal laboratories. In his view, the federal government has a number of basic research laboratories involved in biological research, for instance those of the NIH; it also has laboratories involved in testing and surveillance, such as those of the NTP. The NCTR fills a gap between these two sorts of laboratories.

As examples of recent activities of NCTR, Hart cites development of microencapsulation to be used in lieu of gavage in bioassays. The techniques being developed will be used by NCI and NTP, and they will also be available to laboratories in the private sector. As another example, NCTR has developed a software package so that NTP's contract laboratories can transmit their data and observations to NCTR in a standard format. The data and observations can then be called up from the NCTR computer by either NTP or the laboratory that reported it.

Hart himself is very interested in the question of the validity of the carcinogenicity bioassay. Although all human carcinogens (except arsenic and benzene) have been shown to cause cancer in animals, only a few have been tested in the "standard bioassay" [27]. Hart is discussing carrying out a systematic review of the standard bioassay with the objective of determining its predictive value as compared to the predictive value of animal tests in general. He would also like to make a systematic examination of the effects of different routes of exposure on carcinogenicity of a small number of substances.

The most famous study done by NCTR is almost certainly the "megamouse study" or ED_{01} (for effective dose to cause tumors in 1% of the 23,000-plus exposed mice). The study showed that the well-known animal carcinogen, 2-acetylaminofluorene, caused both liver and bladder tumors [4,28]. Interestingly, the dose response curves for the two tumors differed significantly: the incidence of liver tumors increased almost proportionally to dose while the incidence of bladder tumors increased very little at low doses, and the dose response curve was much more of a "hockey stick" in shape than a straight line. The results of ED_{01} provided so much information that NCTR organized a workshop to discuss it. Scientists from all sectors of the economy attended, and the meeting allowed interested persons to advance their interpretations and have them heard by their peers [29].

In October 1983, at the request of the White House Office of Science and Technology Policy, NCTR held a consensus workshop on formaldehyde. Formaldehyde poses a regulatory problem for the federal government; the Consumer Products Safety Commission acted to ban the use of formaldehyde in some products, but a court sent the regulation back to the Agency for reconsideration. In November 1983, the EPA announced that it was considering regulation. As of December 1983, OSHA had decided not to alter its current exposure standard. The NCTR workshop, which brought together scientists from industry, government, labor organizations, environmental organizations, and universities, considered the available evidence and tried to arrive at consensus about the toxicity of formaldehyde. Consensus was reached on many technical issues, but not on the level of carcinogenic risk posed by formaldehyde. In other words, the technical step closest to the regulatory act was not taken.

Despite the failure to achieve consensus on the risk of formaldehyde, the NCTR-hosted workshop provided a test of this approach for evaluating data that are being considered in the regulatory arena. It must be judged at least a partial success. It seems appropriate that NCTR, which is dedicated to problem solving, was at the center of an effort to integrate scientific data and opinions in a thorny regulatory issue.

B. Estimating Carcinogenic Risks

Every federal research and regulatory agency that has responsibility in the area of carcinogenesis prepares risk assessments. In particular, EPA, CPSC, and OSHA estimate the number of people at risk from specific exposures to justify their regulatory activities. As the preambles of the proposed regulations has increased in length in the *Federal Register*, those agencies have published more information about the procedures they use. They will not be discussed in this chapter. Instead, this section will mention one opportunity for sharpening risk assessment tools and an importance advance in techniques to estimate carcinogenic risks quantitatively.

1. The Use of Structural Activity Relationship Analysis at the EPA

The new chemicals program under the Toxic Substances Control Act (TSCA) requires that a manufacturer or importer of a chemical that is not present in commerce notify the EPA at least 90 days before manufacture or import is to begin. The notification is to include certain information about the new chemical, including any available toxicity data. About half of the notifications contain no toxicity information [30], and in many of those cases, EPA staff make estimates of the potential toxicity by comparing the structure of the new chemical to those of existing chemicals of known toxicity.

The EPA staff who make these decisions are daily accumulating experience with the mechanics of structural activity relationship analysis. In their collective experience are many examples of their being sure about the validity of the analysis and others in which they had to "swallow uncertainty" to come to a decision. Early in 1984, EPA announced plans to carry out some short-term tests on some "new chemicals" that have already been reviewed to determine if additional information would have altered decisions made without it.

2. Improving Information About the Shape of Dose Response Curves from Bioassays

One difficulty inherent in using data from bioassays to estimate human risks is that the dose response curve provides little or no data about the shape of the curve between the last data point and zero dose. This is especially a problem in a bioassay that measures cancer incidence or mortality in 100 animals; tumor frequencies much below 10% are difficult to measure. At the same time, we are vitally interested in how many cancers will be produced by doses 1/100, 1/1000, or 1/10,000 times smaller, and the information available from the bioassay gives no guidance [4].

D. Hoel et al. [31] have reviewed the literature about the possibility of using adducts between test chemicals (or their metabolites) and DNA to estimate the shape of the response curve at lower doses. In short, since carcinogens interact with DNA, they expect that measuring the kinetics of binding between the suspected carcinogen and DNA will be predictive of the dose response at doses too low to be measured in the bioassay. They also point out that the adduct formation measurements can be precise enough to yield other information that is impossible to obtain from bioassays. For instance, a chemical may bind at different sites on DNA. Binding at one chemical site may be associated with carcinogenicity; at other sites, it may have no effect. They refer to one paper which showed that that was indeed the case. Therefore, when enough information is available the DNA adduct formation studies can separate those interactions which are associated with carcinogenicity for other interactions.

Importantly for public health, these studies allow more accurate estimates of risk. Also importantly, for economic considerations, in (probably) every case the refined measurement will reduce the risk estimate.

C. Identifying Cancer Risks in Human Populations

1. Epidemiology

The only certain information about *human* cancer is that obtained from studies of humans. Structural activity relationship analysis, short-term tests, and animal tests allow predictions to be made about the likely effects of a substance on human beings. But, because of differences in genetics and metabolism, we cannot be certain of the human effects.

As everyone knows, ethical considerations forbid testing substances for carcinogenicity in humans, and therefore, studies of human cancer rely on making observations of populations known to be or suspected to be exposed to carcinogens or that are experiencing unusual cancer rates. Many substances have never been tested for carcinogenicity, and most that have were tested as single substances. Humans encounter bewildering mixtures of carcinogens that no laboratory testing can mimic. So one important aspect of epidemiology is that it can detect human risks that have not been predicted from animal studies and probably cannot be.

A frequently cited difficulty with epidemiology is that it can find carcinogens only after people have sickened and died. There is nothing to be done about that criticism. However, that is no reason not to do epidemiology. Unexpected findings are possible also. The reduced cancer rates seen in some populations are important to the current interest in the possibility of dietary factors reducing cancer risks.

National Cancer Institute (NCI). The NCI has been active in attempts to identify geographic clustering of cancers across the country. Observing unusual rates of cancer can result in hypotheses about possible associations between exposures, including occupational exposures, and cancer. For instance, in 1975 NCI published the famous "cancer maps" that showed higher than usual rates of lung cancer and mesothelioma in the Tidewater area of Virginia. Subsequent investigation associated the higher rates with employment in shipyards (and probably with exposure to asbestos). In 1982, a study showed that excess lung cancer in eastern Pennsylvania was associated with work in the steel industry. This study suggests that other tasks besides coke oven operations in steel mills may be associated with elevated lung cancer risks [1].

Not occupationally related, but interesting, the cancer maps showed that white women living in the South were at higher risk of oral cancer than women living in other sections of the country. Additional studies showed that excess risk was associated with dipping snuff. Given the current advertising of snuff as an alternative to cigarettes, the study deserves wide publicity. As stated by Doll and Peto [3], there seems to be no use of tobacco without added cancer risk.

The NCI maintains the Surveillance, Epidemiology, and End Results (SEER) program that collects information about cancer incidence, mortality, survival rates, and cancer trends. There are now ten designated SEER centers, and their coverage of the population is sufficiently representative to allow determination of cancer rates in subgroups of the national population—whites, blacks, American Indians, Hispanics, Hawaiians, Filipinos, Chinese, and Japanese. Although there are problems with interpreting incidence data from the SEER program [3], the data provide our best estimate of what is happening to cancer incidence in the country.

The *1983 NCI Annual Plan* [1] cites studies of occupationally exposed groups as a valuable means to identify chemical and physical carcinogens. The Institute states that it plans to expand efforts directed at studying occupational carcinogens. One area receiving emphasis will be studies of occupationally related cancer in minority groups.

National Institute for Occupational Safety and Health (NIOSH). NIOSH conducts studies of occupational diseases and also collects data about exposures to hazards in the workplace. With the great interest in dioxins during the past few years, NIOSH has established a registry of workers who manufactured chemicals in which dioxins are produced as byproducts. Examination of the health of that group of workers will be important to learning about the human effects of the chemicals. Other registries have been established for workers who were exposed to beryllium, kepone, and other specific substances.

2. Data Systems Useful for Epidemiology

A role unique to the federal government is the ability to collect information on samples of the nation's population. These national data collections already play an important role in epidemiology, and certain programs recently established and considered for the future are making the data more useful.

Three types of information are useful in assessing the carcinogenic risk of a substance or understanding the factors that contribute to cancer rates in a study population. The three types of information—(1) health status, (2) exposure information, (3) physical, chemical, and biological properties of substances—are collected within different departments of the federal government.

Information about health status. The Department of Health and Human Services (HHS) is primarily responsible for administering health data collection, storage, and analysis projects. An overview of HHS programs, as well as other departments' health data collection activities, can be found in *Selected Topics in Federal Health Statistics* [32].

The National Center for Health Statistics (NCHS) collects information on natality (from birth certificate information reported to the Center by the states), mortality (from death certificate information reported to the Center by the states), marriage, and divorce. In addition to collecting vital statistics, NCHS conducts several general purpose surveys about the health of the U.S. population [33].

The Health Interview Survey (HIS) is the principle source of information on the health of the civilian noninstitutionalized population of the United States. Each year, approximately 40,000 households containing 120,000 persons are sampled to provide data on a range of health measures, including the incidence of illnesses and accidental injuries, the prevalence of diseases and impairments, the extent of disability, and the use of health care services.

The Health and Nutrition Examination Survey (HANES) collects and uses data from interviews and physical examinations to estimate the prevalence of chronic diseases, establish physiological standards for various tests, determine the nutritional status of the population, and access exposure levels to certain substances. Both HANES I (1971–1975) and HANES II (1976–1979) examined approximately 20,000 persons.

The white cell count levels determined in HANES I were used for comparative purposes in an epidemiologic study of laboratory workers exposed to toxic chemicals. HANES II gathered information about dietary intake of substances which have been associated with lower cancer risks—vitamins A and C, and with higher cancer risks—fats.

Mortality followback surveys conducted by NCHS are an efficient means to augment the information routinely reported in vital records. The efficiency for eliciting additional information about deaths is related to the relative rareness of death as an event in the U.S. population. About 1% of the population dies annually, and cancer-related deaths are reported for about 20% of the 1% or a total of about 0.2% of the entire population. The followback studies sample directly from the relatively small file of death certificates of interest. Follow-up surveys were conducted annually from 1961 through 1968, but then discontinued because of NCHS's lack of resources. The surveys of 1966–1968 focused on smoking [33].

NCHS is planning a national mortality followback survey for 1985 [33]. It will investigate (1) associations between risk factors and deaths from preventable causes, (2) health care services provided to older people in the last year of life, and (3) socioeconomic differentials in mortality. The possible associations addressed in (1) will be explored by making mail inquiries of the person who provided the funeral director with information to be included on the death certificate. In the earlier surveys, the response rate was about 90%.

NCHS responded to a recommendations that occupational mortality data could be important in planning disease prevention efforts by examining the information about occupation and industry included on death certificates. About 90% of 5000 death certificates chosen at random contained sufficient information to allow coding of occupation and industry according to the Census Bureau's Alphabetical Index of Industries and Occupations. With funding and cooperation from NIOSH, NCHS has organized training courses, and 15 states have begun coding occupation and industry on death certificates so that all entries will be consistent with the Census Bureau coding used for surveys and censuses. This will greatly facilitate epidemiologists' use of death certificates to obtain information about industry and occupation.

A recent, very useful innovation from NCHS is the *National Death Index (NDI)*. Deaths in the United States are registered by the states, and records are transmitted on microfilm or tape to NCHS for compilation into national data. Historically because there was no integration of records for the country as a whole, no mechanism had existed at the national level to determine if a person had died. Since 1981, the NDI has provided a single source of information about deaths in the United States.

When an investigator supplies the NDI with a minimum set of identifiers, generally the person's name and social security number or date of birth, the NDI can tell whether or not the person has died and which state holds his death certificate. The investigator can then contact the state for the death certificate. Previously, the investigator would have had to contact each state separately to determine if the person had died. The National Cancer Institute intends to use the NDI to determine the fact of death for all persons who are entered in a SEER registry. This use is expected to reduce the number of people whose deaths go unrecorded and to improve SEER's information about survival times after cancer is diagnosed and treated.

Exposure information. Between 1972 and 1974, NIOSH conducted the National Occupation Hazard Survey (NOHS) to provide estimates of the proportion of employees exposed to potential health hazards in various industries. More recently, it has repeated the survey, now called the National Occupation Exposure Survey, and the results of that survey are expected to be available in 1984.

The Environmental Protection Agency (EPA) is the lead agency in the regulation of chemicals. However, many studies have been critical of its data collection about exposures. The general impression is that the efforts are incomplete and have generated data of limited usefulness [4].

Information about chemicals. Information about carcinogenicity of substances is produced by industry and government laboratories. It is generally disseminated by publication in scientific journals or government reports, and as may be too often the case, such dissemination may be ineffective. The NTP now publishes an *Annual Report on Carcinogens* which brings together information derived from the World Health Organization's International Agency for Research on Cancer, from the scientific literature, and from federal laboratories.

Data systems for epidemiology. Through various departments and programs, the federal government collects data of the three kinds necessary for epidemiologic inquiries into cancer incidence and mortality. The data systems are not what everyone wants. For instance, some people would like NDI to hold copies of death certificates so that investigators would not have to take the additional step of having to approach the state that holds the record. However, our federal records system requires substantial changes to make it possible. Despite still present drawbacks, improvements have been made and efforts are being made to improve the use of the systems [34].

From time to time proposals have been made to allow health researchers to link federal record systems together to facilitate epidemiology [4,35]. The idea is attractive to many researchers. For instance, linking together information collected about an individual in HANES with information about him at the Social Security Administration and, perhaps, the Veterans Administration would provide a great deal of information about work history and socioeconomic status, all of which are important in evaluating risk factors. Such a system is not without peril. Those who object to it see it putting too much information together about individuals. At this time, although linkage systems are still discussed, there is no apparent movement toward setting up such systems. Only partly joking, some experts have commented that 1984 is not a good year to erect a system that would tie together and allow access to many records about an individual.

IV. PROPHYLAXIS EFFORTS

Smoking causes more cancer than any other single activity (Chapter 1), and it interacts with some occupational exposures to increase cancer rates [3,4,36]. The Public Health Service has high-lighted the importance of smoking by publishing *The Health Consequences of Smoking: Cancer* [36]. The reasons for recent decreases in smoking among U.S. males are not clearly understood, but the publicity about its adverse health effects has surely contributed to that change.

In recent years a growing body of evidence has drawn attention to the possibility that components of the diet may contribute to cancer occurrence or prevention [3-5]. In cooperation with the National Heart, Lung, and Blood Institute of the NIH, NCI is sponsoring a massive trial of the effects of supplementing the dietary intake of beta-carotene. The study involves more than 20,000 male physicians, and it will investigate the hypothesis that consumption of beta-carotene is associated with reduced cancer incidence.

V. GOVERNMENT POLICY OFFICES

Both the executive and legislative branches of the government recognize that the employees of the research and regulatory agencies are sometimes so caught up in their jobs that they cannot step back and evaluate what they have done and how they might modify what they are doing. To provide evaluation and policy review mechanisms, both branches of government call upon the National Academy of Sciences, and both have set up science and technology review and assessment offices.

A. The National Academy of Sciences

The National Academy of Sciences (NAS), through committees organized around single topics, has commented on almost every aspect of federal research. For instance, the NAS was asked to review the National Cancer Plan that was formulated to guide the recently enlarged NCI in the early 1970s [37]. It has commented on general aspects of federal carcinogen testing policy and on specific programs dealing with pesticides and, in particular, with some bothersome chemicals such as saccharin.

For some years, discussions have gone on about possible alternatives to the present federal policies about making decisions about carcinogens. In response to that interest, the NAS [38] produced a document recommending changes in the federal risk assessment policy. That document has been greeted with approval by many observers and, if it is implemented, promises to change the federal government's risk assessment policies.

B. Office of Science and Technology Policy

The Office of Science and Technology Policy (OSTP), located in the Executive Office of the White House, advises the President. It made an important contribution to the discussion about federal cancer policy in a 1979 paper [39]. That paper made implicit the notion that making technical decisions about whether or not a substance is a carcinogen appropriately belongs to scientists; decisions about regulating carcinogens are better made by other people in the regulatory agencies. In 1982, OSTP released a draft report that purported to review recent advances in the understanding of carcinogenesis and, based on those changes, suggested altering the framework of federal government decision making about the carcinogenicity of substances. The paper was roughly criticized, as often happens to drafts; was revised at NCTR and published for comment in the *Federal Register* in May 1984.

The Office of Science and Technology Policy was the organizing factor behind the formaldehyde consensus workshop that was hosted by NCTR. In recent years, OSTP has produced papers and facilitated discussion of important subjects pertaining to carcinogens. To some extent, it appears to be concerned with issues right at the juncture of research and policy. That is where it should be.

C. Office of Technology Assessment

The Office of Technology Assessment (OTA) is a staff office of the U.S. Congress. Since 1977 it has been involved in commenting on policies relating to cancer. In that year, Congress asked it to review the scientific evidence about the carcinogenicity of saccharin. The *Assessment of Technologies for Determining Cancer Risks from the Environment* [4] marked its first assessment devoted to a single topic in environmental health. That assessment and the more famous Doll and Peto paper [3] produced on contract as input to it discuss the proportion of cancers that are associated with various human activities. Among other things, that assessment argued for the execution of a large scale trial of beta-carotene and for large case-control studies of the most common cancers to better pin down risk factors. A 1983 report, *The Role of Genetic Testing in the Prevention of Occupational Disease* [40] discusses the possible applications of cytogenetic testing to screening for precancerous conditions.

In addition to studies directed at cancer or occupational diseases, other OTA reports (for a complete listing, contact Publishing Office, OTA, Washington, D.C. 20510) describe the potential for various technologies to impact health. Cancer is discussed in many of the reports.

VI. SUMMARY AND CONCLUSIONS

This chapter has focused on positive highlights of the federal research efforts directed at cancer. It has not pointed out criticisms. For instance, many observers damned the "cancer virus program" at NCI because it spent millions of dollars over a period of 30 years and did not find a virus until 1981. In fact, had it not been for advances in immunology and recombinant DNA technologies, the search might still be without success. Nevertheless, basic research into the biology of tumor viruses that accompanied the search produced much of the information important to the recent spectacular gains in understanding cancer.

Almost at the other end of the scientific spectrum from molecular biology is the federal government's collecting data about health status, exposures, and properties of chemicals. Those data are critical for studying populations of people to understand what is important to developing or avoiding cancer.

The support of basic research and the collection of data on a national level are probably best done by the federal government. The recent advances in both areas argue that the government's policies can be fruitful.

Additionally, the efforts to decide what is a technical issue of risk assessment and what is a policy issue of regulation have produced important discussions of the roles of scientists and regulators. One way or another, the government is involving experts from all sectors of society in discussing the best ways to decide what substances are carcinogens. Those discussions and the resolutions of them do not have the heady excitment, nor the upbeat sense of progress that swirl around understanding cancer genes, but they are an important aspect of the federal government's research directed at reducing the toll of occupational cancer.

REFERENCES

1. National Cancer Institute. *National Cancer Program: 1982 Director's Report and Annual Plan, FY* 1984–1988, National Institutes of Health, Bethesda, MD, 1983.
2. Office of Technology Assessment, United States Congress, *Controls for Health and Safety in the Workplace.* Government Printing Office, Washington, D.C., in press, 1984.
3. R. Doll and R. Peto, The causes of cancer: Quantitative estimates of avoidable risks of cancer in the United States today, *J. Natl. Cancer Inst. 66*:1191-1308 (1981).
4. Office of Technology Assessment, United States Congress, *Assessment of Technologies for Determining Cancer Risks from the Environment*, Government Printing Office, Washington, D.C., 1981. [reprinted as *Cancer Risk: Assessing and Reducing the Dangers in our Society*, Westview Press, Boulder, CO, 1982.]
5. B. N. Ames, Dietary carcinogens and anticarcinogens, *Science 221*: 1256-1264 (1983).
6. J. D. Watson and F. H. C. Crick, A structure for deoxyribose nucleic acid, *Nature 171*:737-739 (1953).
7. F. Crick, The double helix: A personal view, *Nature 248*:766-769 (1974).
8. J. D. Watson, *The Double Helix*, New American Library, New York, 1969.
9. H. O. Smith, Nucleotide sequence specificity of restriction endonucleases, *Science 205*:455-462 (1979).
10. O. T. Avery, C. M. MacLeod, and M. McCarty. Induction of transformation by a deoxyribonucleic acid fraction isolated from *Pneumococcus* type III, *J. Expt. Med. 54*:137-146 (1944).

11. M. Gough, S. Lederberg, Methylated bases in the host-modified deoxy-ribonucleic acid of *Escherichia coli* and bacteriophage lambda, *J. Bacteriol. 91*:1460–1468 (1967).

12. W. Arber, Promotion and limitation of genetic exchange, *Science 205*: 361–365 (1979).

13. Office of Technology Assessment, United States Congress. *Impacts of Applied Genetics*, Government Printing Office, Washington, D.C., 1981.

14. Office of Technology Assessment, United States Congress, *Commercial Biotechnology: An International Analysis*, Government Printing Office, Washington, D.C. in press, 1983.

15. J. Maurice, Human 'T' leukemia virus still suspected in AIDS, *J. Am. Med. Assoc. 250*:1015–1021 (1983).

16. R. A. Weinberg, The secrets of cancer cells, *The Atlantic 252*(2):82 et. seq. (August 1983).

17. R. A. Weinberg, A molecular basis of cancer, *Scientific American, 249*: 126 et. seq. (1983).

18. H. Land, L. F. Parada, and R. A. Weinberg, Tumorigenic conversion of primary embryo fibroblasts requires at least two cooperating oncogenes, *Nature 304*:596–602 (1983).

19. H. E. Ruley, Adenovirus early region 1A enables viral and cellular transforming genes to transform primary cells in culture, *Nature 304*:602–606 (1983).

20. J. Cairns and J. Logan, Step by step into carcinogenesis, *Nature 304*: 582–583 (1983).

21. R. F. Newbold and R. W. Overell, Fibroblast immortality is a prerequisite for transformation by EJ c-Ha-*ras* oncogene, *Nature 304*:648–651 (1983).

22. M. W. Hunkapiller and H. N. Antoniades, Human platelet-derived growth factor (PDGF): Amino-terminal amino acid sequence, *Science 220*:963–965 (1983).

23. R. R. Doolittle, M. W. Hunkapiller, L. E. Hood, S. G. DeVare, K. C. Robbins, S. A. Aaronson, and H. N. Antoniades, A simian sarcoma virus *onc* gene, v-*sis*, is derived from the gene (or genes) encoding human platelet-derived growth factor, *Science 221*:275–276 (1983). And in "Research News" in the same issue: J. L. Marx, *onc* Gene related to growth factor gene, *Science 221*:248 (1983).

24. M. Bishop, Talk delivered at the Congressional Workshop on 'Carcinogenesis—From the Environment to the Gene.' Banbury House, Cold Spring Harbor Laboratory, November 19–21, 1982.

25. L. G. Hart, J. E. Huff, J. A. Moore, and D. P. Rall, The National Toxi-

cology Program's Research and Testing Activities, *Hazard Assessment of Chemicals 2*:191-244 (1982).

26. National Toxicology Program. *Annual Plan for Fiscal Year 1983*, Department of Health and Human Services, Washington, D.C., 1983.
27. J. M. Sontag, N. P. Page, and U. Saffiotti, *Guidelines for Carcinogenic Bioassay in Small Rodents*, National Cancer Institute, Bethesda, MD, 1976.
28. *J. of Environmental Pathol. and Toxicol. 3*:(3) (1980) (Entire issue).
29. D. H. Hughes, R. D. Bruce, R. W. Hart, L. Fishbein, D. W. Gaylor, J. M. Smith, and W. W. Carlton, A Report on the workshop on biological and statistical implications of the ED_{01} Study and related data bases, *Fundamental and Applied Toxicol. 3*:127-160 (1983).
30. Office of Technology Assessment, United States Congress, *The Information Content of Premanufacture Notices*, Government Printing Office, Washington, D.C., 1983.
31. D. G. Hoel, N. L. Kaplan, and M. W. Anderson, Implication of nonlinear kinetics on risk estimation in carcinogenesis, *Science 219*:1032-1037 (1983).
32. Office of Technology Assessment, United States Congress, *Selected Topics in Federal Health Statistics*, Government Printing Office, Washington, D.C., 1979.
33. National Center for Health Statistics, *Data Systems of the National Center for Health Statistics*, Department of Health and Human Services, Hyattsville, MD, 1981.
34. H. Rosenberg, New research directions on socioeconomic differentials in mortality: United States of America, Paper presented at UN/WHO/CICRED Network on Socio-Economic Differential Mortality in the Industrialized Societies, Rome, May 24-27, 1983.
35. G. W. Beebe, Long-term follow-up is a problem, *Am. J. Public Health 73*:245-246 (1983).
36. Surgeon General, *The Health Consequences of Smoking: Cancer*, Department of Health and Human Services, Rockville, MD, 1982.
37. Office of Technology Assessment, United States Congress, *Technology Transfer at the National Institutes of Health*, Government Printing Office, Washington, D.C., 1982.
38. National Research Council, *Risk Assessment in the Federal Government: Managing the Process*, National Academy Press, Washington, D.C., 1983.
39. Office of Science and Technology Policy, *Identification, Characterization, and Control of Potential Human Carcinogens: A Framework for*

Federal Decision-Making, Executive Office of the President, Washington, D.C., 1979. Also in *J. Natl. Cancer Inst. 64*:169–176, (1980).

40. Office of Technology Assessment, United States Congress, *The Role of Genetic Testing in the Prevention of Occupational Disease*, Government Printing Office, Washington, D.C., 1983.

5

THE ROLE AND IMPACT OF INDUSTRIAL HYGIENE EXPERTISE IN REDUCING CANCER RISKS

Howard L. Kusnetz*
Shell Oil Company
Houston, Texas

Jeremiah Lynch*
Exxon Chemical Company
East Millstone, New Jersey

I. INTRODUCTION

Industrial hygiene is traditionally defined as, "that science and art devoted to the recognition, evaluation and control of those en-

---

*Formerly Engineering Director, U.S. Public Health Service. (Retired.)

99

vironmental factors or stresses arising in or from the workplace, which may cause sickness, impaired health and well-being, or significant discomfort and inefficiency among workers or among citizens of the community" [1]. To this, possibly in recognition of the need for knowing the unknown, the concept of "anticipation" of health hazards has been proposed [2].

Even this simple view of industrial hygiene is not universally understood. Goelzer, of the World Health Organization, notes, "In many countries, both industrialized and developing, industrial hygiene as we know it and practice it, simply does not exist as a science in its own right. In others it exists, but more in theory than in practice" [3]. The industrial hygienist has been charged with the responsibility, "(1) to recognize the environmental factors and to understand their effect on man and his well-being; (2) to evaluate, on the basis of experience and with the aid of quantitative measurement techniques, the magnitude of these stresses in terms of ability to impair man's health and well-being; and (3) to prescribe methods to eliminate, control or reduce such stresses when necessary to alleviate their effect" [1]. Thus, the industrial hygienist must be attuned to the vast range of subtleties relating workplace exposure and infirmity. Toxicology, pharmacokinetics, oncology, genetics, teratology—the sciences as well as the words—today must be part of the hygienist's working knowledge.

II. INDUSTRIAL HYGIENE: HISTORIC ROLE AND MODERN PRACTICE

In a practical world the industrial hygienist provides a bridge between the medical and biologic sciences and operations in the workplace. This required range of knowledge makes the tasks of control and prevention of occupational disease in general, and occupational cancer in particular, very difficult.

At one time it was common for the disciplines of toxicology and industrial hygiene to be combined in the same person. Now, as biologists extend their knowledge back to the molecular level and industrial hygienists forward through the engineering phases of control, individuals combining the full range of skills are rare. Biologists and industrial hygienists need jointly to convert the whole range of available biologic evidence about a material into a quantitative basis for risk control. For carcinogens, this risk assessment process [4] starts with the evidence on the causal linkage of a chemical with a cancer, and proceeds through dose-response and exposure assessments to a characterization of human risk with attendant uncertainty. The risk estimate is then used by the industrial hygienist as a starting point for risk control decisions. The biologist and the industrial hygienist work together to define and reduce uncertainties so as to be able to make sound control decisions.

For a better perspective of the industrial hygienist's role, it would be useful to review briefly the evolution of industrial hygiene as a profession. Historian Jacqueline Corn looks at three distinct time periods, pre-OSH Act*, in which there were major changes in direction, emphasis, or policy in industrial hygiene practice. These are 1900-1917, 1935-1949, and 1969-1970 [5].

Corn views the first period as one in which the problems of industrial health and safety had "become a crisis of epidemic proportions which demanded attention." The diseases which commanded the most attention included plumbism, mercurialism, silicosis, and phosphorus poisoning.

Occupationally induced cancer did not command much attention. In fact, the major attention was not on disease, but on accidents and industrial safety. Two landmark events characterized the period. The Triangle Shirtwaist fire of 1911 focused attention on the appalling safety conditions in the "sweatshop" industries of the time, and in 1914 the Federal Office of Industrial Hygiene and Sanitation was established. That office evolved into the National Institute for Occupational Safety and Health (NIOSH).

Corn's second period, 1933-1946, encompasses a time of increased social legislation in the United States. The Social Security

---

*The Occupational Safety and Health Act, signed into law on December 28, 1970, and effective four months later. The acronym, "OSHA" is generally taken to mean the Occupational Safety and Health Administration (of the U.S. Department of Labor).

Act of 1935 included provisions to make federal funds available
for grants-in-aid to states for industrial hygiene work. Soon, state
units of industrial hygiene, which were generally in the labor departments of a handful of states, proliferated in the health departments of most states. The stage was set for increased emphasis and
interest on health effects in the workplace—among them, occupational cancers.

Corn cites 1969 as the entry year to the next, modern, stage of
industrial hygiene, presumably because 1969 saw the start of the
91st Congress which eventually passed the OSH Act. In fact, in
1966 President Johnson saw the need for a national attack on occupational diseases. Presidential Assistant Joseph Califano created
a three-man team to review the national needs and to recommend
legislation: Deputy Presidential Science Advisor Ivan Bennett;
safety expert Floyd Van Atta, representing the U.S. Department
of Labor; and industrial hygienist Howard Kusnetz, representing
the U.S. Department of Health, Education and Welfare. A comprehensive document, "A Federal Program for Occupational Health
and Safety," which became the basis for the OSH Act, emerged.
Four years later the Act was signed into law. It is interesting to
note that the study team put "health" before "safety" in the report title. Congress, recognizing perhaps that safety hazards were
much easier to understand, reversed the two.

Since 1970, industrial hygiene has grown rapidly. Membership
in the American Industrial Hygiene Association increased from
1600 in 1971 to more than 6000 in 1983. The distribution of
certified industrial hygienists in the workforce in 1982–1983
is also illuminating (Table 1). From 1982 to 1983, there was a
13.4% increase among all certified hygienists. In 1983, about two-
thirds of all certified industrial hygienists were in the private
sector with 62.2% in industry and 6.4% as private consultants.
Current hard data on the academic backgrounds of industrial hygienists are not available. It is evident, however, from speaking
with the secretaries of the professional associations and a review of
the directories that the majority of practicing industrial hygienists
are not engineers. The lack of engineering background increases
the difficulty of the industrial hygienists's ability to solve the technical problems of prevention and control.

Table 1 Distribution of Certified Industrial Hygienists (CIH) by Employer, 1982 and 1983

	1982		1983	
	No.	%	No.	%
Industry	1063	63.5	1184	62.2
U.S. government	258	15.4	299	15.7
State and local government	101	6.0	116	6.1
Foreign	18	1.1	30	1.6
Academicians	150	9.0	170	8.9
Labor	9	0.5	10	0.5
Consultants	56	3.3	87	4.6
Other	20	1.2	7	0.4
Totals	1675	100.0	1903	100.0

Source: Roster of Diplomates of the American Board of Industrial Hygiene, 1982 and 1983.

The well-qualified industrial hygienist, capable of dealing with the complex problems of industrial carcinogenesis, possesses a varied mix of skills. Industrial hygienists, like physicians or engineers, are practitioners who use science as a tool in their efforts to reduce the chance of harm to people who work. An industrial hygienist needs to know the chemistry and physics of health hazards, the biology of health effects, the engineering principles of manufacturing and hazard control, and such related skills as ergonomics, psychology, and management. While most industrial hygienists have one or more areas in which they specialize (e.g., acoustics, industrial ventilation, aerosol physics), all are expected to have a working knowledge of the whole range of skills required to manage risks, starting from before they have been clearly identified through their eventual control and beyond.

The industrial hygienist has the major task of identifying materials and their uses in the workplace, of determining the probability of disease resulting from exposure, and of devising methods to ensure that the probability of exposure-related disease becomes vanishingly low. To do this and to take part in the risk assessment/ risk management process, the industrial hygienist must be able to demonstrate how the suspect materials, *in use*, will have sufficient contact potential so that there is reasonable possibility of disease occurring.

The process through which industrial hygienists reduce risk better describes what they are than does a list of skills they use. The industrial hygienist must evaluate the work environment to discover who is at risk, where the suspect carcinogen is present, who else could be exposed, how often workers are exposed, and what the patterns of exposure are. Workers move around, production processes and work practices change, and the concentration of a substance in air will vary widely over time and space. Statistical sampling strategies must be used to allow decisions of known accuracy to be made in spite of the many variables in the workplace. The truth must not only be found, it must be seen to be found, so that the evidence will convince management to take possibly expensive risk reduction actions. Sound inferential statistics with low error require adequate numbers of samples.

In the past, industrial hygiene has been hampered by cumbersome sampling and analytic techniques which severely limited the number of measurements which could be made. Modern monitoring techniques using solid sorbents in place of liquid-in-glass samplers, passive samplers instead of pumps, and automatic instrumental analysis in place of wet chemistry have made it possible to make the number of measurements needed for reliable decisions. In the future we can look forward to the development of computer based automated monitoring systems coupled with worker tracking systems which together allow real time, multisubstance, automatic exposure measurement.

Professional industrial hygiene today is more than taking atmospheric or breathing-zone samples. It encompasses the entire spectrum of the industrial process. The potential for exposure is first raised when management contemplates producing a product. The physical properties (gas, liquid, solid), conditions under which the product will be manufactured (temperature, pressure), materials of construction and their reactions with raw materials, intermediates, and final product, and the points at which the process is necessarily opened to human contact (e.g., quality assurance sampling, product loading), all contribute to the potential for exposure.

The best way to achieve reliable, cost-effective control of health hazards is to build hazard controls into each plant when it is initially constructed. Retrofitting controls to an existing plant is more expensive and interferes with production. Once the design basis has been determined, the choice can be made of emission control options which are appropriate to the toxicity or potency of any hazardous chemicals present. Certain detailed matters such as exhaust hood designs are best reviewed in the final design. Personal protective equipment would be a last stage of control specified in the operating manual for the finished plant.

Properly, the industrial hygienist is actively involved through the pilot plant and semiworks stages. During construction the industrial hygienist should check on control of construction and start-up hazards. When the plant is finally built, there should be good knowledge of how exposures can occur. Effective training of the workers in the unit becomes a necessary tool for control. It is only when the plant is running that the requirements for regular and routine atmospheric monitoring occur. Even at this point, consideration of the atmosphere alone is insufficient to determine risks or to prevent effects.

The industrial hygienist must consider all the routes of entry of contaminants to the body. Ingestion may occur through contaminated hands, improper storage of lunches, chewing gum, chewing tobacco, candy, or cigarettes. It may occur when an operator licks his finger to turn the page in a procedures manual or when a dispatcher wets the tip of his pencil with his tongue. Unprotected coffee cups, sugar bowls, and spoons for stirring coffee may be the vectors of exposure by ingestion. Skin absorption occurs when the contaminant is soluble in body surface fluids, or when solvents carrying potential carcinogens penetrate the skin.

Breaks in the skin are frequent and inevitable routes of entry for contaminants. Slow-acting materials may find entry through the unbroken skin when they are permitted to remain in intimate contact through contaminated clothing. Scrotal cancers seen in some European machinists are attributable to oil-soaked coveralls and poor personal hygiene.

There are habits or cultural factors which may be different for each work force. Is it the usual practice to take samples of products for home use? Are solvents available for personal clean-up? Does potential for exposure exist from contaminated work clothing brought home by other family members? Is personal hygiene of such a nature that exposure is likely to occur by other than direct workplace contact? Constant investigation and knowledge of such factors are necessary for defining fully the extent of the potential for real risk.

One stark and tragic effect of personal habits on cancer induction appeared in a recent report on the continuing studies of radium dial painters. The *Wall Street Journal* noted [6],

> Women at the plant sometimes painted their fingernails with radium paint "for kicks," says Pearl Schott, who worked as a dial painter here from 1946 to 1977. Others took pots of radium paint home and painted light switches so that they would glow in the dark. They routinely contaminated their hair, arms, legs and feet with the radioactive material accidentally while they worked, and they wiped paint-covered hands on the front of their work smocks.
>
> Mrs. Schott had breast cancer and a mastectomy in 1964. Afterward, she returned to work, still unaware of the possible hazard. She developed more tumors on her feet and now walks with a cane. "If they'd have warned me," she says, "maybe I'd have had the good sense to get out."

Clearly, one vital phase of the industrial hygienist's job is to see that the message does get to the employees.

III. INTERPRETING DATA

If it were true that any one contact with a carcinogen necessarily leads to cancer, sampling would need only to show the presence or absence of the suspect agent. Professional sophisticated analyses and evaluations would not be needed. Exposure to carcinogens, however, leads only to a probability—not a certainty—of cancer. Cancer rate tends to rise with level, frequency, and duration of exposure. How this happens differs from one carcinogen to another. The concept of the threshold limit value (TLV) is a more useful one, being indicative of the potential for harm and, therefore, the potential for control. Understanding and properly using the TLV is part of the industrial hygienist's daily concerns.

The term "threshold limit value" is a trademark of the American Conference of Governmental Industrial Hygienists (ACGIH). The ACGIH defines TLVs: "Threshold limit values refer to airborne concentrations of substances and represent conditions under which it is believed that all workers may be repeatedly exposed, day after day, without adverse effect" [7]. Given that cancer potential depends on many factors, the concept of daily or repeated exposure being necessary for probable manifestation of the disease becomes the driving force in the protocols which the industrial hygienist prepares for evaluating the environment.

The operative words in the definition of the TLV are, "day after day." The reality is that relatively long periods of exposure at some low value may, in fact, cause cancers. This is in distinction to the regulatory dictum that any exposure exceeding some arbitrary, legally mandated value at any time is improper. The legal value is set on the theory that even in the absence of acute, massive exposures, those which exceed a properly established allowable level on any one day are sufficient to cause disease. For noncarcinogens, such a theory almost certainly does not apply. For most carcinogens, the theory may not apply either. Thus, to set up sampling protocols the industrial hygienist must consider the variations of atmospheric exposure. He must set his sampling protocols so that daily, diurnal, weekly, monthly, and seasonal variations of exposure are taken into account. The industrial hygienist must look not only for the worst case, that is, where leaks or emissions are likely to occur, but at all aspects of workplace use of potential carcinogens. He must know what the exposure is, or is likely to be, throughout each workday. It is improper to evaluate known periods of exposure and arbitrarily to postulate or assign zero exposure to certain non-work periods. Coffee breaks, bathroom visits, and lunch hours do not necessarily carry with them zero exposure. The extrapolation from short exposure times to full work days is frequently performed improperly. One example of such an incorrectly performed extrapolation and analysis was illustrated with regard to reputed ethylene oxide exposure in Finland [8].

Ethylene oxide had been shown in other studies to have caused cancers such as peritoneal mesothelioma and mononuclear leukemia in rats [9]. In November 1982, a study was published by K. Hemminki from the Institute of Occupational Health in Helsinki concerning the possible effect of increased spontaneous abortions in hospital sterilizing staff.

Hemminki studied spontaneous abortions in hospital staffs in Finland for the years 1973–1979. In his concluding paragraphs he stated, "Ethylene oxide concentrations have been measured in many sterilising units in Finnish hospitals; 8-hour weighted mean concentrations have ranged from 0.1 to 0.5 ppm with peak concentration up to 250 ppm . . . The present findings indicate the exposure to ethylene oxide in hospitals correlates with and increased frequency of spontaneous abortions."

The inference from these statements is that the measurements were related to the exposures of the women in whom the abortions were studied, especially in view of the unequivocal statement of 8-hour time weighted averages. In February 1983, a group of American health experts, including a certified industrial hygienist, visited Finland and the author. The conclusions in their report make interesting reading. They state [10]:

> While the authors do not directly claim that EtO TWA_8 exposures of 0.1 to 0.5 ppm are those for women in the study, this inference is made. Specifically, *no exposure level data were collected for the study* (emphasis added). The reader of the study report article may be led to believe that these exposure values are ones that cause an increased risk of spontaneous abortions.

The authors also noted that no exposure measurements were made as a part of the study. Almost all the industrial hygiene measurements were made after the study was completed. The limited number of grab-type samples were not TWA_8 measurements. A nonvalid procedure (by OSHA and ACGIH guidelines) was used in calculating the reported TWA_8 values published in the study.

Clearly, improper methods for obtaining exposure data and improper interpretations of data can invalidate and make useless a health study such as this.

Properly performed industrial hygiene analyses are vital for epidemiologic studies. The occupational epidemiologist seeks to discover associations between factors in the work environment and disease. Such associations are useful because when combined with confirmatory evidence they may point to cause and thereby make prevention possible. A difficulty all epidemiologists encounter is that while exposures to chemical substances may be the likely causes of occupational carcinogenesis, the extent of exposures is seldom known. Instead, epidemiologists must use surrogates such as employment in a chemical plant or work in a particular job. Using such surrogates, excesses of cancer are sometimes seen, but the agent at fault is not identified so risk reduction measures are hindered if not prevented altogether.

To improve exposure classification, epidemiologists have asked industrial hygienists to construct retrospective exposure histories for workers or groups of workers. This very difficult task is often attempted because of the potential value of the result. Typically, the epidemiologist and industrial hygienist will divide a cohort into job title or homogeneous exposure groups and attempt qualitatively to describe exposure by some simple scheme (high, medium, or low) at various periods of time over the history of the plant. Judged by the logical conclusions reached in some such studies, it appears that the results may be usable, but they are scientifically unsatisfying because independent verification is not possible. Even when done well, retrospective exposure estimation deals inadequately with the excursions and episodes which may be determining factors in disease occurrence. The specific exposure histories of those affected and of those in control groups are, ideally, what is needed. Yet all too often they are not available.

As an example of the misuse of retrospective exposure evaluation, we illustrate the case of the benzene standard. In 1977 OSHA published an Emergency Temporary Standard (ETS) for benzene, followed by a permanent rule. The basis for the risk assessment which led to the ETS and the rule appeared to be a paper by Infante [11]. This study concerned two rubber hydrochloride plants in Ohio with benzene exposure. Exposures were estimated by assuming they had fallen within the recommended limits at that time. Data, admittedly, were quite inadequate for one of the plants and even worse for the second plant where, at the time of the study, there were no environmental data. Nevertheless, assumptions as to environmental conditions were made.

In follow-up papers by Rinsky [12] and by White [13], some additional environmental analyses were made. Some very limited information was available for industrial hygiene assessment of the second plant. Operations were conducted in that plant, according to White, from 1949 to 1965. Some data were published by Rinsky, but are identified only as follows: "The only environmental data available from this plant are shown in Table IX [NIOSH 1977] believed to be taken around 1957. The exact date is uncertain." Of interest is that there is no indication that the employees in whom cancer was detected worked at any of the tasks cited, or whether there was any relation between the very sketchy data supplied in the NIOSH report and Rinsky paper and the workers' exposures.

In the paper by White et al., the assumption of exposure was maintained. White stated, "For this risk assessment, we assumed that exposures were at the recommended standard for that time. We recognized that some workers may have been exposed occasionally to higher levels. However, we believe that the average exposure experience for the entire study population *is adequately represented by the levels in Table I*, (emphasis added) and that the use of these levels actually may have overestimated benzene exposures for many workers." The table cited is an historic review of recommended environmental levels for 8-hour time weighted average benzene concentrations between the years 1937 and 1975. However, the table carries a footnote which makes its validity questionable. The table states that the recommended benzene level during the years 1937–1940 was 150 ppm. The footnote states: "No recommended level was available before 1941."

Assumptions made in this series of studies are probably inaccurate, cannot be relied upon for adequate exposure estimates or for risk assessment, and are likely to lead to misleading conclusions.

Various schemes have been developed for retrospective exposure estimates. We have noted the use of recommended or standard values by Infante et al. Other techniques include measuring exposure of selected members of homogeneous exposure groups; qualitatively estimating exposure on a simple scale; and linking inventory with job location data to obtain subjective estimates of the "could have/could not have been exposed" type.

An elaborate procedure for retrospective exposure estimates was found necessary in a specific case at the company of one of the authors (Kusnetz). It is presented here in some detail to show the depth of investigation which may be necessary, and to serve as a guide for those contemplating their own exposure estimate studies.

A study of death certificates had indicated a statistically significant increase in acute myelogenous leukemia (AML) at one petroleum refinery, and a nonstatistically significant increase at a second. Benzene has been manufactured at both locations for a quarter century or so. (Benzene is reputed to increase the rate of AML.) The question was whether a *direct* link between AML and benzene could be established. Initial examination failed to link the individual cases to obvious exposure. Since some of the affected employees had started work as far back as the 1920s, and since sufficient industrial hygiene monitoring data before the 1970s did not exist, some effort had to be made to estimate the early exposures. The technique used comprises the following major tasks to reconstruct pertinent benzene-related information.

Task (a) is performed first. Task (b) depends on the results of (a). Tasks (c) and (d) may begin concomitant with (a). The work products of each task group become tools for the panel performing the historic exposure study. Personnel selected for each work group have work experience at the location dating as far back as possible. Retirees are especially valuable in the process. The tasks are: (a) Conduct process reviews for units containing benzene to establish startup/shutdown dates and major process or operating changes; (b) identify benzene related jobs and tasks which could result in benzene exposure (e.g., opening process equipment, gauging tanks) by frequency, duration, and sensory description; (c) identify benzene-related work practices to determine if and how benzene was used and would not necessarily be identified in (b) (were personal protective equipment or other measures used to minimize exposure?); and (d) develop occupational personal histories of diagnosed leukemia cases using service records and interviews (while the primary emphasis is on potential benzene exposure, information on other possible exposures is also solicited).

An historic anecdotal exposure study is then performed separately and approximately concurrently at both locations. The tools provided to each panel are the work products of the earlier tasks. The panels act to reconstruct the historic benzene exposures for all benzene-related jobs at their respective locations.

Finally, using the product of the several tasks, the workplace benzene exposures for diagnosed leukemia cases can be assessed to the extent that any retrospective assessment is possible.

An added useful feature of a retrospective exposure study is to conduct structured experiments quantitatively to determine actual benzene exposures for typical work practices as identified earlier.

It is evident that there really are two major areas for understanding and assessing risk due to industrial carcinogens. For the industrial hygienist, the first is to review, retrospectively, what may have existed and to make the best possible estimate. The second is to so develop sampling and environmental evaluation protocols that future exposures—short-term as well as time weighted average long-term—are measured properly and are recorded together with a detailed analysis of the work environment and work practices of each individual employee.

Of more importance, however, is the need to ensure that in the future these retrospective studies will no longer be necessary. Farsighted corporations today are attempting to capture as much information as possible with regard to employee exposure. By the end of the century, that is, when at least two decades for cancer latency have passed, occupational cancers which may be manifest may then be identifiable with their proximate causes.

There is one anomaly, however, in industrial hygiene practice which may render even such a careful procedure invalid. The prime function of the industrial hygienist is to prevent occupational disease and infirmity. He must be sure that controls are in place and working. Industrial hygiene sampling in well-run establishments, therefore, is usually geared to "worst-case" situations. That is, the industrial hygienist pinpoints those areas where escape of contaminants into the environment is likely to occur. Emphasis is on sampling in these high potential areas. If and when a leak does occur, environmental samples are usually taken while the equipment is being repaired or the situation is being corrected. The values derived from the sampling and analytic protocols are likely to be high because of the nature of the situation. In any event, over time there may be a disproportionate number of samples from areas where exposure is known or suspected to be high. Routine samples under normal conditions may be fewer and further apart in time. A distorted picture of real exposure may be built up over a 10- or 20-year period of data gathering.

To the extent that some diseases, including some cancers, may be caused by peak exposures, even for short periods of time, "worst case" data are valuable. However, if diseases and cancers are caused by long-term exposures to low or moderate levels, the "worst case" emphasis is insufficient for fully relating cause and effect. It is necessary, therefore, to sample, at least on a preplanned and periodic basis, those areas of the work environment where nothing is going wrong, but where the employees spend much of their time.

IV. CANCER PREVENTION

The risk posed by an occupational carcinogen could be eliminated by banning the substance and thus completely preventing exposure. This is an easy health solution but one which may have other serious adverse consequences. The challenge in industrial hygiene is to devise means by which even the most hazardous materials can be manufactured and used safely. Of course, safe operations with potent carcinogens are expensive and the economics may make a suitable substitute attractive. In many instances, however, the usefulness of a material is great enough to justify the high cost of stringent control. The case of the control of the potent carcinogen bis chloromethyl ether (BCME) is an illustration of what can be done when available industrial hygiene controls are applied.

A. The Bis Chloromethyl Ether Experience

Building on aerospace experience, a high degree of safety is achieved through the use of several overlapping, redundant layers of control. The following measures, which are a composite of those used by several BCME manufacturers, illustrate the principle.

1. Containment

In completely closed processes no exposure can occur. Closed processes become open where there are leaks and where they are deliberately opened as for product sample collection. Each potential emission source such as pump and agitator shaft seals, valve stems, flanges, or vents, is analyzed for ways to reduce emissions. Mechanical seals are used instead of packing glands. Vents, where unavoidable, are provided with scrubbers. Samples are collected using closed containers and closed sampling loops.

2. Ventilation

When some release may still occur, local exhaust ventilation is used. Exhaust systems capture and remove any contaminants from the workplace before anyone is exposed.

3. Isolation

Control areas which contain all BCME production and consumption operations are maintained under negative pressure so that airflow is always from outside to inside. Entrance is restricted to essential workers. Since operations are remotely controlled, only inspection and limited maintenance require entry.

4. Personal Protection

To prevent the dispersion of BCME by contaminated work clothing, operators change into special clothing when entering the controlled area. Operators also use either supplied air respirators with associated protective clothing or a full air-pressurized suit. Upon exiting the controlled area, the operator showers after placing protective clothing in a water-filled container.

5. Monitoring

In addition to personal samples, area measurements with installed automatic monitoring systems give real time, instantaneous indications of a rise in BCME concentration in air which would indicate a leak or other inadvertent release.

B. Research

Industrial hygiene, because of its unique position as a bridge between the biological sciences which identify and define health effects and the physical sciences and engineering which effect control, has a key role in research planning. The research is either done directly by the industrial hygienist or in collaboration with the related disciplines of medicine, biology, and epidemiology. Of all the scientifically sound studies which might be done, some make more valuable contributions to the overall process of reducing risk than others. It is helpful to view the studies and actions needed to control cancer risk in a typical occupational setting, as a collection of information-generating and hazard-control events occurring in sequence or in parallel. As an aid in planning, such events could be charted by common engineering planning techniques. Looked at in this way, it is possible to see which studies and actions are needed, which are on the critical path so that their timing determines the timing of the overall project, and how to assess the value of each piece of information or control action so as to achieve cost optimization. The industrial hygienist who, in a bridge role, is best able to see from one end of the process to the other has the perspective to do this planning.

Some specific industrial hygiene research activities illustrate this point.

1. Epidemiologic Cohort Studies

The exposure ranking provided by industrial hygiene was discussed earlier. With this exposure information, the epidemiologist can identify and confirm (or deny) an occupational carcinogen by identifying (or not) the existence of exposure or dose response, even qualitatively.

2. Clinical and Case Control Studies

Cohort studies are rarely quantitative enough to yield dose-response relationships. Studies which look at small groups of cases and controls can make use of intensive exposure data to arrive at dose-response estimates.

3. Toxicologic Research

In animal experiments the dose should be administered by the routes and in the time patterns which mimic human exposure in order for these experiments to have the best chances of modeling human health effects insofar as these aspects are concerned. Further, the significance of the wide variations in exposure, which are common in the workplace, can best be interpreted by pharma-cokinetic studies which follow the time course of a carcinogen and its metabolites through the body. Such studies may discover that only peak dose rates above a threshold have effect, and this fact would have enormous implications for monitoring and control. Indicating what the shape of the dose- or exposure-response curve might be as doses or exposures decrease is, too, quite valuable.

4. Monitoring Methods Development

Even though it is recognized that at times health effects data must drive sampling and analytic methods development, eventually one must be able to measure exposure in order to be able to control. Further, given the wide variability of exposure and the variety of workers exposed, statistical sampling strategies which achieve optimum trade-off between cost and error are needed for reliable decision making.

5. Control Methods Development

The fundamental consideration in occupational carcinogenesis control is the set of measures taken in the workplace to reduce risk. Engineers expert in plant and process design use the specialized skills of industrial hygienists in the less familiar field of health hazard control. Traditional industrial ventilation technique development has long been led by the American Conference of Governmental Industrial Hygienists. More recently, research into contaminant release patterns and related mathematical modeling in chemical process industries has made it possible to predict exposures in plants not yet built. To back up these engineering measures personal protective equipment of known effectiveness is also provided and used. Respirators and clothing are tested against each specific carcinogen. Advances in respirator technology which increase protection and acceptance are being pressed. Lastly, behavioral studies of how to persuade workers to make better use of protective equipment are joint efforts of industrial hygiene and behavioral scientists.

V. INDUSTRIAL HYGIENE WORLDWIDE

The practice of industrial hygiene as described here applies to the United States and approximately to the United Kingdom, Canada, and Australia where the profession is well developed and established. Elsewhere in the industrialized nations these functions are partially performed by others (physicians, engineers, technicians). Goelzer of the World Health Organization notes that in the developing countries they may not be performed at all [3]. From the point of view of a multinational company seeking to maintain health protection for all its employees worldwide, these differences must be considered in implementing industrial hygiene programs. Other cross-cultural differences are management attitudes and perceptions. Some managers may have not yet come to grips with the realization that we probably cannot achieve zero risk for carcinogens. Further, in some countries the concept of assumed risk of certain occupations gets in the way of risk reduction programs.

Worker knowledge is also a variable. In some countries the understanding of health hazards on the part of workers and the general public is rudimentary. The development of training programs which achieve a balanced understanding of health risks so as to encourage precautionary measures without causing alarm requires a sensitive appreciation of worker attitudes and beliefs.

Industrial hygiene has been an evolving profession. To the extent that it can translate the jargon of the biologic world for the managers and workers who would be exposed, and to the extent that it can help the cancer researcher understand the "real world" where exposure may occur, industrial hygiene becomes an important factor in preventing occupationally induced cancers. It is, indeed, the bridge between the health-related sciences and the front line where reduction and prevention of cancer incidence takes place.

REFERENCES

1. *1982-1983 Membership Directory*, American Industrial Hygiene Association, Akron, OH.
2. Ralph Langner, Private Communication to President, AIHA.
3. B. I. F. Goelzer, The practice of industrial hygiene in other countries, *Annals of the American Conference of Governmental Industrial Hygienists*, ACGIH, Cincinnati, OH, 1983, pp. 25-31.
4. National Research Council, *Risk Assessment in the Federal Government: Managing the Process*, National Academy Press, Washington, D.C. (1983).
5. J. K. Corn, Historical review of industrial hygiene, *Annals of the American Conference of Governmental Industrial Hygienists*, ACGIH, Cincinnati, OH, 1983, pp. 13-17.
6. Bill Richards, The dial painters, *The Wall Street Journal (Southwest Edition)*, *LXXII*:55, page 1 (September 19, 1983).
7. *Threshold Limit Values, 1983. American Conference of Governmental Industrial Hygienists*, Cincinnati, OH (1983).
8. K. Hemminki, P. Mutaner, *et al.*, Spontaneous abortions in hospital staff engaged in sterilising instruments with chemical agents, *Br. Med. J. 285*: 1461-1463 (20 November, 1982).
9. W. Snellings, C. Weill, and R. Maronpot, Final report ethylene oxide two-year inhalation study on rats. *Report 44-20*, Bushy Run Research Center, Pittsburgh, PA (Jan. 1981).

10. An Assessment Report of: K. Heminki, et al., Spontaneous abortions in hospital staff engaged in sterilizing instruments with chemical agents, *British Medical Journal, 285*:1461-1463. (Nov. 20, 1982). (Ethylene Oxide Industry Council, Washington, D.C. May, 1984).
11. P. F. Infante, R. A. Rinsky, J. K. Wagoner, and R. J. Young, Leukemia in benzene workers, *Lancet ii,* 76-78 (1977).
12. R. A. Rinsky, R. J. Young, and A. B. Smith, Leukemia in benzene workers, *Am. J. of Ind. Med.* 2:217-245 (1981).
13. M. C. White, P. F. Infante, and K. C. Chu, A quantitative estimate of leukemia mortality associated with occupational exposure to benzene, *Risk Analysis* 2:195-204 (1982).

6

AN ILLUSTRATION OF VOLUNTARY ACTIONS TO REDUCE CARCINOGENIC RISKS IN THE WORKPLACE

Bruce W. Karrh
E. I. du Pont de Nemours and Company
Wilmington, Delaware

I. INTRODUCTION

A commitment to the well-being of every employee is the back-
bone of an effective occupational safety and health program.
Many major corporations in American industry, including Du
Pont, know that the value of that commitment lies not in words,
but in actions which demonstrate the commitment. And many
companies have had substantial programs in place much longer
than there have been governmental requirements to have them.

Du Pont is one such company, but before focusing on Du Pont's
voluntary actions with regard to reducing carcinogenic risk in industry, some background on the company's overall approach to
health and safety is necessary. Du Pont, not atypical of industry,
serves as an example of what has and what can be done.

The safety and health of employees have been of prime importance to Du Pont since the company's founding in 1802. The
company's founder, Eleuthere Irenee du Pont understood two
things quite well: first, how the volatile nature of his product—
black powder—necessitated protective measures to ensure the
safety and health of employees; and second, the value of his
workers' lives. He felt personally responsible for his employees,
and in his earliest rules (1811) and regulations, made it clear that
management is directly responsible for establishing and maintaining safe and healthful workplaces.

For example, Mr. du Pont prohibited employees from entering a
new or rebuilt mill before management entered to assess the risk
to safety or health. Further, he lived on-site, beside the mills with
his employees, in order to have direct interaction with daily operations and demonstrate his commitment. This kind of commitment
has evolved through successive generations of management. For
nearly 200 years, the Du Pont Company has refined and improved

it, effecting change not through reaction to external concerns, but through initiatives based on internal dedication and concern. It is Du Pont's conviction that all accidents are preventable and all identified health risks are containable.

II. MEDICAL PROGRAM DEVELOPMENT

In the early 1800s, the medical surveillance program began with Mr. E. I. du Pont's retaining Dr. Pierre Didier to provide a form of occupational medicine for his employees. Those with work-related problems were treated by Dr. Didier who charged Mr. du Pont for the service. Personal services were billed to patients.

In 1915, a more formal medical surveillance program was initiated. The company's Executive Committee charged competent doctors with the responsibility of performing annual physical examinations for all employees. The Committee also appointed a full-time medical director to oversee this medical program which was aimed at discovering and remedying organic troubles or diseases.

The next year, Du Pont's first site hospital was built at Parlin, New Jersey, by the plant's doctor. At the same time, departmental safety commissions began collecting safety performance data.

Du Pont's safety and health initiatives continued to expand at a rapid pace. In 1925, routine chest x-rays were included as part of employee physical examinations. The next year, a corporate safety and fire protection division was created, and safety audits of sites across the company were instituted.

In 1935, Haskell Laboratory for Toxicology and Industrial Medicine was built. As one of the first such institutions in industry, its mission was to explore the risks associated with chemicals to which employees were exposed. Among other medical program developments, Du Pont began including audiometric tests as part of employee physicals in the 1950s, and in 1956 established a formal epidemiology program which includes a cancer registry. Further, in 1977, an occupational health survey group was established to audit plant industrial hygiene practices. Two years later, Du Pont began to computerize the exposure tracking system to document employee work and exposure history. In 1980, occupational medical program surveys were started. One of the most recent advances was the company's extending the alcoholism program to retirees and to employees' families and survivors. At present, Du Pont is initiating a health improvement program to help employees stay healthy and live longer, fuller, more productive lives.

III. CARCINOGENIC RISK

The history of the company's effort in assessing carcinogenic risk begins in the early 1930s when the first cases of bladder cancer which could be attributed to occupational factors were diagnosed at Du Pont's Chambers Works in Salem County, New Jersey. Dye workers were involved. With this discovery, Du Pont began cystoscopic examinations of dye workers as part of an ongoing program to protect workers and to study the situation. A full-time urologist was hired to conduct these examinations, and industrial protective measures were undertaken, such as the installation of forced ventilation.

Du Pont took its findings and actions to the public. Du Pont, in cooperation with Memorial Hospital in New York, sponsored a Symposium on Anilin Tumors of the Bladder. Dr. Gerhmann, the company's medical director, delivered a paper providing an overview of Du Pont's study, its findings, and the examination procedures [1]. Presentations at the symposium contained the first public incrimination of betanaphthylamine, alphanaphthylamine, and benzidine as suspected carcinogens.

To further the study of bladder cancer and to formalize investigation into occupational health, Du Pont's Executive Committee recommended the establishment of Haskell Laboratory. And through the mid-1930s, publications concerning the company's bladder tumor experience continued, including those by Dr. Victor D. Washburn [2] and Dr. G. G. Gerhmann [3]. The company's chief pathologist, Dr. Wilhelm Hueper, along with two other Du Pont doctors, published a paper in the *Journal of Industrial Hygiene* in 1938 identifying betanaphthylamine as a carcinogen in laboratory animals and the most likely cause of bladder cancer in the dye workers.

Recognition and action with reference to bladder tumors and the eventual discontinuance of the production of betanaphthylamine and the production and use of benzidine taught Du Pont that producing chemicals was not unlike our earlier manufacture of black powder—both included the presence of hazards, the only difference being how the hazard presented itself. This awareness served to reaffirm a strong commitment to occupational safety and health, a commitment that persists and is the basis for Du Pont's current program.

IV. INTERNAL ACTIVITIES

Internal activities to control carcinogenic risk in the workplace include seven comprehensive program components, all of which represent what can be done by corporations on a voluntary basis. These activities, as carried out in Du Pont, are: toxicological testing; hazard detection; hazard determination procedure for carcinogenic risk; medical surveillance programs; occupational medicine; epidemiology surveillance; specific epidemiology studies for cancer.

A. Toxicological Testing

To determine the toxic properties of chemical compounds and the precautions required to use them safely is the primary objective of Haskell Laboratory for Toxicology and Industrial Medicine.

Haskell tests about 500 substances a year. While many short-term tests are used to identify potential carcinogenic compounds, increased emphasis has been given to designing and using long-term tests. This necessitated three expansions in the laboratory in the last 15 years, and the staff increased from 9 in 1935 to over 240 in 1983.

The types of tests include (1) short-term or acute studies to determine the inherent toxicity of a substance and to establish a baseline for further work (the tests involve oral, inhalation and dermal/ocular studies), (2) subacute studies to determine if a material produces cumulative effects and what organ or organs are primarily involved, and (3) long-term animal tests to determine whether a chemical can cause chronic toxicity. These take several years to complete. Recognizing human carcinogens is difficult because 20 years may pass between the initial exposure to a carcinogen and the appearance of a cancer. Further complications can occur from a lack of an exact correlation between animal and human carcinogens.

Short-term assays or "screens" supplement Haskell's effort to provide a relatively prompt and inexpensive indication of possible carcinogenicity. Such assays measure the ability of compounds to cause mutations, chromosomal damage, or transformation of normal cultural cells to cells that can cause tumors. Haskell was one of the first laboratories to use the *Salmonella*/liver microsome test—better known as the Ames test. This test measures a chemical's ability to induce mutations in bacteria, one indicator of potential carcinogenicity, helping scientists identify substances for more specific testing for carcinogenicity.

Genetic toxicology studies are expanding. In addition to the Ames assay and the Chinese Hamster Ovary test, the sister chromatid exchange assay is used to determine any occurrence of genetic damage. But even with the expanded studies, a need still exists to develop additional assays designed to identify potential mutagens and carcinogens.

Results of our toxicological testing program are encouraging in terms of our ability to recognize toxicity levels and control exposures. Through Du Pont's Acceptable Exposure Limit (AEL) Committee, established in 1978 to lend formality and efficiency to our setting of exposure limits, we have established approximately 300 AELs in the past five years [4].

B. Hazard Detection Program

Detecting hazards often requires a close working relationship between industrial health practitioners, including industrial hygienists, physicians and occupational health nurses, and toxicologists [5]. Du Pont's asbestos disease detection program demonstrates how they interface in an industrial initiative which goes beyond regulation to develop and implement an effective program in a complex area. Du Pont's plant physicians and consultant radiologists performed a comprehensive review of employees/pensioners exposed to asbestos during employment in order to detect early signs of lung abnormalities which would indicate asbestos exposure during employment. Trained plant physicians, nurses and outside radiologists were used to perform the early identification. This was made easier with the help of updated x-ray technology.

The results of our efforts showed that a fraction of one percent of our population had medical abnormalities related to asbestos exposure, and the company has assumed responsibility for any work-related illness or impairment resulting from asbestos exposure.

C.   Hazard Determination Procedure for Carcinogenic Risk

Guidelines concerning hazard determination for carcinogenic or reproductive risk are provided to managers to use in protecting the safety and health of employees, customers, and the public. Originally used in 1975, they have been updated to assure the following objectives are achieved: (1) to ensure prompt assessment of any carcinogenic or reproductive risk from exposure to hazardous chemicals involved directly or indirectly in the manufacture, use, distribution, or disposal of company products, and (2) to ensure development of programs to minimize risk when necessary.

Guidelines are to be followed worldwide and include how hazards are determined, how control programs are developed, and what communication is needed. These procedures supplement any mandatory requirements developed by government agencies for carcinogenic or reproductive toxins. The more stringent limit, either developed by Du Pont or by the national agency, shall apply in each nation.

D.   Medical Surveillance Programs

To assure that Du Pont's sites are maintaining medical programs which reflect corporate standards and practices, occupational physicians from the Medical Division perform medical surveys about every three years. In addition, occupational health surveys are performed by the Safety and Fire Protection Division. The findings help the company strengthen its medical program assets and reorganize in areas which need improvement.

E. Occupational Medicine

Du Pont's routine occupational medical surveillance program was started in 1915 when periodic physical examinations were instituted. It has continued to the present time and includes all employees. Employees receive regular periodic comprehensive physical examinations, which include some tests especially for early detection of cancer, on a frequency determined by age and irrespective of job assignment [5]. In addition, employees who are assigned jobs where there is potential for exposure to hazardous substances may receive more frequent examinations and/or additional special tests. For example, employees who work where there is potential for exposure to hexamethylphosphoramide (HMPA), an animal carcinogen, receive annual examinations irrespective of age.

Pensioned former employees are eligible to continue receiving the comprehensive physical examination annually, with the results being sent to his or her personal physician for the use of the pensioned former employee.

F. Epidemiology Surveillance Program

Begun in 1956, the company's epidemiology surveillance program was one of the first of its scope in industry. One component is entirely devoted to cancer epidemiology in response to the intensified concern over carcinogens as new chemical substances are produced and used [6].

The cancer program has two objectives: first to measure cancer incidence and mortality among employees and mortality among pensioners; and second, to identify company sites that have a significant excess of any type of cancer and determine if the excess may have occurred as a result of exposure to a substance in the workplace.

To help assure that the objectives are met, the cancer surveillance program includes: (1) routine reporting of cancer cases among employees and cancer deaths among employees and retirees, (2) maintenance of a cancer registry in which employee cancer incidence is recorded, (3) routine collection of population statistics by age, sex, and payroll class for all company locations to provide a population base for statistical analyses, (4) periodic analyses of cancer incidence in plants, offices, and laboratories; and (5) cohort studies to investigate cancer morbidity and/or mortality among persons who have worked with materials which have been suspected or known carcinogens, like dimethyl sulfate, formaldehyde, acrylonitrile, and others.

Du Pont has developed a system for identifying and controlling carcinogens. Consequently, the company has acted upon more than 30 substances in addition to the 19 for which specific OSHA rules are applied. Such are controlled below exposure levels where adverse effects may occur. Supplementary actions include employee notification, external communication where appropriate, reviewing medical and exposure histories and, if necessary, restricting sales of a product. A computer-based system was installed in 1979 to improve Du Pont's employee exposure data access and retrieval capability. Called the Personal Environment Record System (PERS), it stores, records, and reports individual employee work assignments and exposures to various chemicals [5].

G. Specific Epidemiology Studies for Cancer

The most important type of epidemiological cancer research conducted in the company is cohort studies, which focus on employees who have worked with known or suspected carcinogens. The cancer incidence or cancer deaths of the cohort are then compared with the experience of another population. Several cohort studies have been completed or are under way—DMS, chloroprene, acrylonitrile, and benzene [7–11].

Another type of study which can be done is case-control studies, such as studies of persons exposed to formaldehyde. These studies were done to determine whether occupational exposure to

formaldehyde increases Du Pont workers' risk of developing
cancer, with special attention to cancers of the lung and upper
respiratory tract, particularly the nasal cavities. The case-control
study of cancer mortality surveyed workers exposed to formaldehyde for 1957–1979. In none of the analyses was formaldehyde
workers' relative risk of cancer significantly greater than 1.0.
There were no nasal cancer deaths and no lung cancer excesses.
Findings suggested that cancer mortality rates in the company's
formaldehyde-exposed workers were no higher than rates among
nonexposed workers.

V. EXTERNAL ACTIVITIES

External initiatives are an integral part of industry's collective effort to help control carcinogenic risk in the workplace. Such initiatives represent a collective approach, built on the expertise, experiences, and good will of all industries, the government, and technical and professional organizations.

Notable collective industry efforts in which Du Pont is also
involved include the Chemical Industry Institute of Toxicology
(CIIT) and the American Industrial Health Council (AIHC). Interaction with governmental regulatory agencies includes the development of the Toxic Substances Control Act (TSCA), the Environmental Protection Agency (EPA), and the Occupational Safety
and Health Administration (OSHA).

A. Chemical Industry Institute of Toxicology

The Chemical Industry Institute of Toxicology (CIIT), Research
Triangle Park, NC, was developed by a concerted effort on the
part of the chemical industry starting in 1974. Du Pont was one of
the 11 founding members of the CIIT with the main purpose of
exploring health effects of chemical compounds and reporting
findings to help answer questions posed by the public, the government, and the chemical industry itself. Over 30 member chemical
companies, representing more than 75% of the chemical industry's
revenues, now sponsor the organization. It is rapidly becoming a
leader in the field of toxicology, and over the next decade its re-

search will focus on understanding the mechanisms by which commodity chemicals may cause a wide variety of toxic effects.

Past research at CIIT has been a significant contributor to what is known about the biological toxicity of chemicals like formaldehyde, toluene, and terephthalic acid, and even ethylene. Their scientific staff have also been researching mutagen and carcinogen causation, liver tumors, cellular responses to chemicals, and reproductive toxicology.

B. American Industrial Health Council

The American Industrial Health Council (AIHC), Scarsdale, NY, was formed as an ad hoc committee within the Synthetic Organic Chemicals Manufacturing Association in 1977 to assist in the development of scientifically sound and economically viable governmental regulation of substances which may cause adverse chronic health effects. The next year it became a free-standing trade association. Virtually all major types of American industries are now represented in the AIHC membership and are in support of the Council's present direction, which involves trying to initiate a national cancer policy for the identification and control of substances which may pose a carcinogenic risk to employees or the general public. The Council is also developing positions on regulatory standards pertaining to other chronic health effects.

C. Toxic Substances Control Act

The membership of the Chemical Manufacturers Association (CMA), Washington, D.C., assisted congress and regulators in the development of the Toxic Substances Control Act (TSCA) [12]. The purpose of TSCA is to assure that existing or new chemical substances which are not otherwise regulated do not present unreasonable health or environmental risks. Since TSCA's inception in 1976, the manufacturers of such chemical substances have primary responsibility for testing them. Federal resources are used to perform or direct testing and related research that is critical to successful regulation, such as assessing hazards about which a small amount of data are available or investigating specific problems for which nonfederal testing is impractical or is not mandated. Such federal programs do not fall entirely under one agency, but the major portion form what is now known as the National Toxicology Program [13].

D. Environmental Protection Agency

The chemical industry has been working in support of the Environmental Protection Agency in many ways. One of the most important efforts concerns the cleanup of hazardous waste sites. Du Pont was one of the first chemical companies to speak out in support of the "superfund" bill of 1980, and since its passage as the Comprehensive Environmental Response, Compensation and Liability Act, the company has worked along with the CMA to promote safe toxic waste disposal.

E. Occupational Safety and Health Administration

A cooperative effort between industry and the Occupational Safety and Health Administration (OSHA) is extremely necessary in establishing and maintaining safe and healthful workplaces. Du Pont and other major companies provided input with regard to the development of many standards, not only those relating to carcinogens, but also other standards including the OSHA Noise Standard and Hearing Conservation Amendment.

Many companies send data relating to potential carcinogens to OSHA and its companion agency, the National Institute for Occupational Safety and Health (NIOSH). A prime example of this kind of industrial initiative is Du Pont's forwarding of research data to OSHA on acrylonitrile. This effort is especially interesting as it represented the first time OSHA accepted data, its interpretation, and recommendations from industry and enacted a regulation based upon this input. OSHA used industry's studies as the basis for development of the acrylonitrile standard. To our knowledge, it is the only OSHA health standard to date (December 1983) that has never been litigated. This latter point is quite important to reducing industrially related cancer in that a health standard which can be applied relatively soon clearly has a good effect contrasted to one which, for any reason, may be delayed or reversed through litigation.

With respect to reducing occupational carcinogenic risk, there is no doubt that there is a recognized need for scientifically based regulations and increased innovation and improvement in controlling carcinogens in the workplace.

VI. SUMMARY

Establishing safe and healthful workplaces requires more than developing a protective philosophy and disseminating policies. And reducing carcinogenic risk requires more than recognizing the need and setting objectives. Keeping employees free from injury and illness requires translating words into actions and policies into programs that work to prevent accidents or diseases.

Industry's effort, as exemplified by the Du Pont program, to control carcinogenic risk in the workplace has been and will continue to be an ongoing commitment, one which the chemical industry pursues to the extent needed, even where it voluntarily goes beyond regulation and exceeds external standards. Du Pont's occupational health program incorporates components specifically designed to focus on carcinogenic risk, and our activities are constantly expanding in the fields of research and workplace procedures and practices to control carcinogenic risk. Along with many in industry, Du Pont does not wait to be regulated where a carcinogenic risk exists, nor does it content itself with compliance, which in the light of new findings, may prove the regulation inadequate.

Further, we know the importance of putting our findings into practice throughout the industry and recognize the value of actively working with governmental regulatory agencies and other organizations to achieve our common goals. Du Pont and many other companies not mentioned due to space constraints, believe much progress has been made in reducing carcinogenic risk in industry and that a sound basis exists for continuing this trend.

REFERENCES

1. G. H. Gerhmann, M.D., *J. Urol. 31*:121 (1934).
2. V. D. Washburn, M.D., *J. Am. Inst. Homeopathy, 29*:9 (1936).
3. G. H. Gerhmann, M.D., *JAMA 107*:143 (1936).
4. C. F. Reinhardt, *J. Am. Coll. Toxicol. 2*:51-55 (1982).
5. J. C. Bonnett, and S. Pell, Du Pont's health surveillance systems, *J. Med. 24*(10):819-823 (October 1982).
6. S. Pell, M. T. O'Berg, and B. W. Karrh, Cancer Epidemiologic surveillance in the Du Pont Company, *J. Med. 20*(11):725-740 (November 1978).
7. S. Pell, Mortality of workers exposed to dimethylsulfate 1932-1974, submitted to American Conference of Governmental Industrial Hygienists and the National Institute for Occupational Safety and Health, 1976.
8. S. Pell, Mortality of workers exposed to chloroprene, *J. Med., 20*:21-29 (1978).
9. M. T. O'Berg, Epidemiologic study of workers exposed to acrylonitrile, *J. Med., 22*(4):245-252 (April 1980).
10. S. K. Hoar, and S. Pell, A retrospective cohort study of mortality and cancer incidence among chemists, *J. Med. 23*(7):485-494 (July 1981).
11. B. W. Karrh, and S. Pell, Brain cancer in the Du Pont Company, *Ann. NY Acad. Sci., 381*:91-96 (1982).
12. 15 USC 2601 et. seq., 1976.
13. *Fed. Reg., 43*(221):53060-53061 (November 15, 1978).

7

A METHODOLOGY FOR REDUCING INDUSTRIALLY RELATED CANCER RISK

Paul F. Deisler, Jr.
Shell Oil Company
Houston, Texas

I. INTRODUCTION

Our knowledge of cancer and carcinogenesis is extensive and grow-ing rapidly. What is still to be discovered, however, is immeasur-ably greater, and our understanding of what is now known is far from complete. Moreover, the uncertainties we face in utilizing data and information from all types of sources to estimate the hu-man risks of cancer from industrially derived agents are so great that the word "uncertainties" is far too mild; a new and stronger word is needed to describe the current state of affairs. Neverthe-less, enough evidence exists from specific cases and from general etiologic studies [1, 2] for it to be clear that risks can exist, that we need to assess them and, where called for, to reduce them.

Protective regulations may not exist for a particular agent or ad-vancing knowledge may indicate that currently existing regulations do not give adequate protection. To improve protection to human health in such instances, it has increasingly become the practice of private firms to set their own standards and thus to lower the risks of cancer (see Chapter 6). For example, in announcing its inten-tion to consider the further regulation of ethylene oxide, the Oc-cupational Safety and Health Administration (OSHA) cited a sig-nificant number of firms which had set their own exposure standards at levels one-tenth of the existing OSHA standard or lower [3].

It is the purpose of this chapter to describe a practical methodology for risk assessment and reduction which is now in use. The methodology takes into account both the incompleteness of our understanding and the aforementioned uncertainties; it therefore offers a way to cope with both problems. Significant aspects of this methodology and its background have been pub-lished or presented elsewhere [4-9]; these aspects will be sum-marized here for the convenience and understanding of the reader in approaching the whole subject. Some new material is included as well.

There are three essential parts to the methodology. The first part is a process whereby information is analyzed, step-by-step and in logical sequence, to determine if a hazard exists, whether it poses risks and, if so, what to do about the risks. The second part is a means for distinguishing between levels of risk to help ensure that the most important risk situations are given priority. This approach will cause the greatest improvements in safety to be achieved for the most people as soon as possible. The third part of the methodology recognizes that risk assessment does not involve only one but rather many scientific and technical disciplines, and especially because of the uncertainties encountered when assessing risks, these disciplines must all be brought to the task in a coordinated manner. In the case of this methodology, it has been found by experience that a core group of representatives of key disciplines plus a knowledgeable chairman, who learn to work consistently with the process and with each other, is essential. Also essential are the following: the willingness of the members of the group to question, and be questioned by, each other; the understanding of the fact that however knowledgeable each may be, each has special knowledge and understanding needed by all; a recognition that others with particular knowledge and understanding need to be consulted by the group, since no group in this complex area can have all requisite knowledge and should not accept inexpert guesses when real knowledge is available; and, finally, it is essential that the chairman be a firm, tactful, patient, articulate, and understanding chairman-facilitator.

II. THE PROCESS OF RISK ASSESSMENT

In the last few years various processes for carrying out risk assessments have been repeatedly described in the literature [10–14]. The principal purpose of each of these processes is to ensure that regulatory agencies consider all relevant and valid scientific and technical information, in as unbiased a manner as possible, to determine whether a hazard to humans is likely to exist, and whether such a hazard poses a significant risk, before deciding whether, how, and to what degree to regulate. The same need for assurance exists within a private firm engaged in evaluating and reducing risks; moreover, the discipline of following a logical process and of sticking to it throughout a risk assessment helps prevent the members of a risk assessment group from leaping ahead in the process and, thus, inadvertently biasing their own scientific judgments by drawing premature conclusions on what the risk reduction actions should be before the need to act is established. The three-stage risk assessment process which forms part of the methodology described in this chapter has been described elsewhere [5, 6] and will therefore only be summarized briefly at this point. As it is summarized, the reader should visualize a risk assessment group in the act of executing the process, stage-by-stage, to the extent needed to reach conclusions at each stage, as well as to reach decisions at each stage, as to whether the process should be continued. A decision that continuation is not warranted and what should then be done is extremely valuable. It helps ensure that rare talents are employed, to the extent possible, only in pursuing important risks.

When the question of risk arises, from whatever quarter, the first stage, *hazard identification*, should be undertaken. In this stage the available data are reviewed to ascertain whether a hazard—the potential to do harm—is identifiable using those data which are found to be valid and relevant. It may or may not, at this early stage, be possible to conclude whether or not an identified hazard applies to humans.

If a hazard is identified, the risk assessment moves on to the second stage, *hazard evaluation*. A full evaluation of the *qualitative* data and the possible relevance of the information for humans where animal test data are used is first made. The data which are most likely to be of use in *quantitative* risk assessment are identified on the basis of this analysis, too, bearing in mind that the mere existence of quantitative data may not justify applying it directly (or after extrapolation) to estimate human risk. The ideal result of this second stage is to be able to describe the ranges of likely responses, qualitative and quantitative, which one might expect if it were possible to test humans under laboratory conditions over a wide range of exposures down to those which humans might possibly encounter in actuality. Clearly, this ideal can only be loosely approximated in actuality, and then only by utilizing a number of assumptions.

With this analysis and with information on actual exposures, a *risk evaluation*, the third and final stage of risk assessment, is now performed. The gathering and assessing of exposure information is essential to establishing risk; a recent study made under the auspices of the National Academy of Sciences [14] rightly identifies this as a distinct activity, *exposure assessment*, which is carried out in parallel with the three sequential decision stages just described.

It is at the end of the third stage of the risk assessment process that the risk is characterized in this methodology by the risk assessment team as *higher, lower*, or, where possible, as *insignificant*. Concluding in which of these risk regions the risk is thought to lie is a final, essential task of the risk assessment group, because the actions required to reduce risk are decided upon depending on the region in which the risk is thought to lie. There is a fourth stage of activity called *risk response*. The risk assessment group can and must assist in this effort, but people familiar with the affected operations must be brought in at this point; these latter people work with industrial hygienists—and others as needed—to determine the most cost-effective ways to respond to and reduce risk.

The setting of risk benchmarks which define the boundaries of the aforementioned risk regions is needed to allow risks to be distinguished from one another. The next three major sections are devoted to this subject.

III. BENCHMARKS FOR RISK ASSESSMENT

Though much of the following discussion deals with quantitative concepts, it is not implied that the elements of quantitative risk assessment should receive heavier emphasis than those of qualitative risk assessment. The quantitative uncertainties are so great that this could hardly be the case in general and, in particular, the reverse may often be true. The clear definition and understanding of the quantitative risk benchmarks and how they are derived is necessary if one is to apply them intelligently. Even when risks have been assessed largely in qualitative terms, this understanding is useful.

A. Measuring Risk

Risk is usually defined as the combination of the probability of a hazard being realized and the factors which describe the magnitude or seriousness of the hazard. In developing the quantitative concepts useful in measuring cancer risk, the focus will be on the probability of occurrence. This probability, p, will be taken as the average probability for individuals in a population under consideration developing *at least* one malignancy in a lifetime over and above any normal, background probability and as a result of exposure to industrially derived agents. This is the principal event to be avoided, and the term "risk" will here refer to this probability.

The variable, p, being dependent on exposure levels, is the primary variable to be measured and, if necessary, reduced by reducing exposures in order to reduce the risk of industrially related cancer. The uncertainties in measuring p are so large, however, that a finely divided risk scale is not meaningful. Even for short extrapolations from the experimental region in animal tests, the existence of an error band as narrow as a factor of ten in p—an order of magnitude—must be considered high accuracy [5]; the same is true for epidemiologic results, largely but not entirely for other reasons. This uncertainty, together with the need to have a sufficient number of risk categories to help set priorities and to indicate the urgencies of action, has led to the aforementioned three risk regions: higher risk (HR), lower risk (LR), and insignificant risk (IR). Consequently, two levels of p are defined: the *level of action* (LOA) which divides HR from LR and the *level of insignificance* (LOI) which divides LR from IR. These two p levels, when quantitatively defined, give as finely divided a risk scale as can be used to report the highly uncertain results of risk assessment.

B. The Level of Insignificance (LOI)

The levels of risk defining which risks are insignificant in individual cases are of great importance to the regulatory community and have been given much thought. The definitions are, for the regulators, not simply based on clear, mathematical conventions, but they depend also on policy considerations, varying legal definitions, or the opinions of courts—in other words, societal factors have entered into these definitions of insignificant risks. Some examples of levels of risk, stated in terms of lifetime probabilities, are these [15–18]: one in a hundred thousand (10^{-5}) as a "target level" for risk for criteria pollutants under the Clean Water Act; one in a million (10^{-6}) for indirect food additives; and zero for direct food additives under the Delaney Amendment of the Pure Food and Drug Act. Indeed, the Supreme Court has stated it would consider the risk of taking a drink of chlorinated water negligible if the risk were one in a billion (10^{-9}), though no time interval was associated with that statement of risk [19].

There seems to be a wide variety of ideas on insignificant risk, starting at about 10^{-5} and going down. From the viewpoint of a private firm, the only practical test for insignificance is statistical. Here, too, even though societal opinion and judgment cannot come into play, the LOI will vary with circumstances. If, for example, a specific exposure situation (SES) such as a specific workplace is considered, the statistically insignificant level of excess risk will vary depending on the background level used for comparison—the local community, for example, or a set of workers not exposed to the agents in question, whether one or more types of malignancies are involved, and how many workers are included in the exposure situation. The same would be true of other SESs of different types (e.g., drinking water from a specific supply, air in a specific locale, etc.), and it is clear that the LOI is specific to the SES under consideration; moreover, the size of the group considered to be subject to the SES affects the value of p which describes the LOI quantitatively. The LOI is, thus, a kind of "group" risk level.

C. The Level of Action (LOA)

The LOI is difficult to determine for each SES. It is also difficult
to know whether the LOI is exceeded or not since as one extra-
polates to lower and lower levels of risk, the large uncertainties in
risk estimation grow larger and larger. For our purposes, too, the
LOI is not the level of risk of first importance since it distinguishes
between LR and IR. Distinguishing between HR and LR has
higher priority in terms of reducing the higher risks first, and establishing the LOA is therefore especially important.

The concept used in this methodology is to set the LOA as a
ceiling on risk, a value *below* which the risk must be made to lie
by monitoring and controlling exposures. The ceiling is set by a
combination of comparative risk, the recognition that there must
be a gap between the LOA and the LOI to define the LR region,
the goal that the contribution of industrially related cancer should
ultimately be markedly reduced from current levels, the reasonable desire that such a contribution should be so small as not to be
determinable with confidence, and the practical need that the
LOA risk levels should not be infeasible of attainment.

Each of the many SESs belongs to a relatively small number of
types of exposure situations (TESs). The TES's are, simply, the
general types of situations leading to exposures: the workplace,
the air we breathe, the water we drink, the additives in the foods
we eat, the medicines we take, and the consumer products we use.
Each TES has its own characteristics of voluntariness of risk acceptance or degree of personal choice or control in taking the risks
which may be involved and, on this basis, a single, separate LOA
can be defined for each TES. The LOAs are therefore few in
number, as used in this methodology, as opposed to the LOIs
which, in principle, can be different for each SES. An LOA, once
defined for a TES, is used for every SES belonging to that TES.
The next section deals with the mathematical definitions of the
LOAs for the various TESs and with the selection of numerical
p values for them.

IV. SELECTING THE LEVEL OF ACTION (LOA)

If possible, it would be useful to set a ceiling value of p for each TES so that, if the actual p values for real SESs are less than the corresponding ceiling values, the ultimate goal of lowering the contribution of industrially related cancer to *below* a selected ceiling contribution would be achieved. Such p values would define the LOAs for the various TESs. Setting such p values is the subject of this section.

A. Basic Relations

Within the population of an entire region such as a country or, indeed, the entire world, each individual is exposed to at least one TES and, frequently, to all. Let the fractions of the population exposed to each TES be $f_1, f_2, \ldots f_i \ldots f_K$, for K total TESs. If in each TES the risk of cancer were *exactly* at the ceiling values, p_{c1}, $p_{c2}, \ldots p_{ci} \ldots p_{cK}$, then the average ceiling probability, $\bar{p}_c$, of industrially related cancer among the entire population would simply be

$$\bar{p}_c = \sum_{i=1}^{K} f_i p_{ci} \tag{1}$$

Here, the p_{ci} values are formal probabilities unrelated to specific causative agents. Thus in calculating $\bar{p}_c$, the p_{ci} values are statistically independent and the products of pairs, triplets, etc., of the p_{ci} for $\bar{p}_c$ (and the p_{ci}) in the low ranges of probabilities relevant for humans are small enough to ignore; Eq. (1) is therefore nearly exact. Given a set of p_{ci} values satisfying Eq. (1) for a given value of $\bar{p}_c$, the average ceiling value of p for any defined population exposed to any set of SESs may be calculated, knowing the fractions of the population in each SES in the set.

It is also true that if F is the fraction of the population which is expected to contract cancer from all causes within the lifetimes of its members, and if g is the fraction of all cancer which is industrially related, then gF is also the average probability of industrially related cancer among the entire population, $\bar{p}$. For $g = g_c$, where g_c is the ceiling value of g, then $\bar{p} = \bar{p}_c$ and

$$g_c F = \sum_{i=1}^{K} f_i p_{ci} \tag{2}$$

Once g_c is chosen, since F is known and the f_i may at least be estimated, there are many sets of p_{ci}-values which can satisfy Eq. (2). How to select appropriate sets of p_{ci}-values will be described later; here and in the next section certain concepts important to utilizing the p_{ci} will be set forth.

The ultimate goal may be expressed in the form,

$$g < g_c \tag{3}$$

which says, simply, that achieving the goal means that the actual average probability of industrially related cancer among the entire population is to be brought to a level *less* than $g_c F$. There are many ways to achieve this. For purposes of practical risk reduction, consider the risk, p_{ij}, defined here as the probability of industrially related cancer in the j-th SES of the i-th TES. If the p_{ij} values for different SES's are statistically independent for all i and j, then the average actual p-value, p_i, for the i-th TES is obtained by summing over j in a manner like that of equation (1), following which Eq. (1), written in terms of $\bar{p}$ and p_i, applies. For this case, then, a practical way to aim toward achieving the goal given by Eq. (3) is to lower exposures so that

$$p_{ij} < p_{ci} \tag{4}$$

for all j and for any i. This is the method of choice, in this methodology, for achieving the goal since it leads to the monitoring, reduction, and control of specific agents in each SES as a practical way to reduce risk. So for any SES, if the actual p value for that SES is lowered by controlling personal exposures to levels below the p_c value for the TES of which that SES is a member, a necessary action has been taken toward achieving the goal as stated by Eq. (3).

B. Coping With Synergism

The actual p_{ij}-values may not act independently because of synergism. Antagonism may also exist; it is, however, a safety bonus and only synergism is of concern. Whether synergism exists or not has no effect on the validity of Eq. (2) or on the values of the p_{ci} selected using Eq. (2), since the p_{ci} are statistically independent as described above and are not related to any carcinogenic agent or agents.

In considering synergism, two cases are of special importance: (a) synergistic action between agents within a particular SES, and (b) synergistic action between agents which, while occurring in different SESs and not in the same SES, affect those individuals who are jointly members of the different SESs involved. The first case is the easier one: so long as the p_{ij} remain independent of each other for all i and j, then whether agents within SES_{ij} interact synergistically or not to produce the value of the p_{ij} has no effect on the applicability of Eq. (4) or, therefore, on our ability ultimately to conform to Eq. (3). Demonstrating the existence of synergism within an SES and determining what levels of exposure will lower the independent and synergistic contributions to p_{ij} so that Eq. (4) is satisfied is a practical difficulty in itself, however.

The second case of synergism is more complex for here Eq. (4) does not apply, given that both sides of the equation are based on statistical independence. In this case, the p_{ij} are no longer independent of each other though the p_{ci} values, of course, are and so they remain as valid control values, though their application to control is now less simple. An example will illustrate this point.

Consider a self-contained region containing a population of n individuals of which n_1 are members of one SES, n_2 are members of a second SES which is itself a member of a different TES than the first SES, and n_{12} are members jointly of both SESs. So,

$$n = n_1 + n_2 - n_{12} \tag{5}$$

Suppose a single agent is responsible for the p_{ij} value in the first SES, where the p_{ij} value is now called p_1 for simplicity, and a different, single agent is responsible for the p_{ij} value in the second SES and, similarly, this p_{ij} value is called p_2. Let p_1 and p_2, which are functions of exposures to the first and second agents, respectively, be the independent responses (probabilities) caused by these agents, and let p_{12} represent the synergistically or jointly caused excess response which is a function of exposures to both the first and second agents together. Without synergism, the goal [Eq. (3)] could be satisfied by

$$f_1 p_1 + f_2 p_2 < f_1 p_{c1} + f_2 p_{c2} \tag{6}$$

where f_1 is the fraction of the n individuals that are in the first SES and f_2 is the same for the second SES. In turn, the chosen way to satisfy Eq. (6) is to satisfy Eq. (4) by setting exposures so that $p_1 < p_{c1}$ and $p_2 < p_{c2}$.

With synergism, one possible equivalent of Eq. (6) is

$$f_1 p_1 + f_2 p_2 + f_{12} p_{12} < f_1 p_{c1} + f_2 p_{c2} \tag{7}$$

where f_{12} is the fraction of the n individuals that are affected by (and members of) both SESs. The simple application of Eq. (4) is no longer possible. However, the selected values of p_{c1} and p_{c2} are used, as before, on the right-hand side of Eq. (7), to set the *combined* risk ceiling for the two SESs.

If Eq. (7) can be put in the form of Eq. (6), thus,

$$f_1 p_1' + f_2 p_2' < f_1 p_{c1} + f_2 p_{c2} \tag{8}$$

then Eq. (4) can be applied in the form

$$p_1' < p_{c1} \tag{9}$$

and

$$p_2' < p_{c2} \tag{10}$$

From Eq. (5),

$$f_1 + f_2 - f_{12} = 1 \tag{11}$$

Combining Eq. (11) with Equations (7) and (8), it is found that with

$$p_1' = p_1 + \frac{f_1 + f_2 - 1}{f_1 + f_2} \, p_{12} \tag{12}$$

and

$$p_2' = p_2 + \frac{f_1 + f_2 - 1}{f_1 + f_2} \, p_{12} \tag{13}$$

expressions (9) and (10) can be satisfied; expression (7) is therefore satisfied also. Thus, even with inter-SES synergism, a case more complex than intra-SES synergism, the criteria embodied in the p_{ci} values may be applied. This simple example can be extended to more SESs, more agents, etc., with similar results.

In practice, the determination of whether synergism exists between two (or more) agents is most difficult. Animal tests are prohibitively large and cumbersome to define the dose-response functions involved for only two agents, and other studies may or may not succeed in detecting synergism. In the usual case, where synergism is unexplored, the simplest control measure is to assume it is absent, to control exposures so that g/g_c becomes as small as it can reasonably be made, and to conduct followup monitoring, surveillance, and epidemiology studies wherever possible to see whether safety goals are being achieved or whether corrections are needed. If risks turn out to be higher than expected, synergism is not the only possible reason. The original risk assessment may prove to be incorrect, an unidentified carcinogen may be present, etc. The same pragmatic approach of making corrections and investigating the matter applies. When the causes of unexpected excess risk are known, this methodology provides a basis for dealing with them, even if synergism is involved.

C. Selecting Numerical Values

The contribution of industrially derived carcinogens to total cancer is now reasonably well known. Thus, for the workplace only, Higginson [1] finds it to lie in the range of 1–5%, whereas Doll and Peto [2] find 2–8% with a preferred value of 4%. Considering the fairly wide uncertainties, these results are in agreement with each other. In both investigations, determining the contributions of such carcinogens in the general environment proved more uncertain still. Adding a very few percentage points to the above figures to yield a preferred value somewhere below 10% for the aggregate contribution of industrially derived carcinogens to total cancer probably characterizes the situation. Given these figures and taking the ranges as statements of the uncertainty of determination of the figures, a choice of g_c of 0.02 or below (2% or less) would constitute a substantial goal for reducing the industrial contribution to cancer to a level difficult to determine. Using a value of 1% (or, $g_c = 0.01$), and since F is approximately 25% (or, 0.25), the left-hand side of equation (2) is known.

On the right-hand side of equation (2), most of the f_i-values are equal to one; that is, most of the population is exposed to most of the TESs with only minor exceptions in such TESs as food additives or medicinal compounds. To assume a value of one for the workplace is excessive, though conservative; for the moment, and acting conservatively, let all the f_i values be one, and let K be six to correspond to the TESs named earlier (see Sec. III, C).

Of the six TESs, most may be considered as largely involuntary in character, with the workplace neither totally voluntary—we must all work somewhere—nor involuntary—a careful worker can exercise significant though not complete control and mitigation over his own exposures. With a 1000-fold (or three orders of magnitude) difference between acceptance of voluntary and involuntary risks [20], a factor of 10 to 100 (or 1 to 2 orders of magnitude) might be applied to distinguish the p_c value for the workplace from the other TESs. To illustrate the principle, a factor of 20 (or 1.3 orders of magnitude) is used.

Considering comparative risk in the workplace, the lifetime risk of death by on-the-job accident for a 30-year worker is about 2.5×10^{-3} [21]. While this hazard is different in many ways from contracting cancer, the seriousness of the latter is high enough to make a comparison reasonable. The Supreme Court has also opined that if regular inhalation yielded a risk of 10^{-3}, a reasonable person might take steps to eliminate or reduce that risk [19]. These observations on more or less comparable risks offer a range,

2.5×10^{-3} down to 10^{-3}, within which p_c for the workplace might reasonably lie—at least when making an initial choice of that p_c value.

With the above considerations, Equation (2) yields a p_c value for the workplace of 2×10^{-3} and, for each of the other five TESs, 10^{-4}. Comparing this latter figure with the aforementioned levels thought to denote insignificant risk (see Sec. III, B) it is seen that it leaves room for the LR region. Moreover, those people exposed to all six TESs have an aggregate ceiling risk of 2.5×10^{-3}.

Of the criteria mentioned in Section III, C for use in selecting p_c values, only one, feasibility, has not yet been considered. Cobler and Hoerger [22] have examined past agency decisions and have estimated the risk levels actually reached after regulation. OSHA's levels exhibit a mode just below 10^{-4}, with other agencies somewhat lower. The distributions of estimated risks are sharply skewed, the means lying below the modes. It would appear that the p_c values, compared with these results, should be feasibly attainable, barring the discovery of some unusually potent carcinogen—a problem which, in any case, would have to be dealt with.

The degree of conservatism introduced by assuming the f value for the workplace to be one is seen by using a value of 0.25, instead, and calculating the resultant g_c. In this case, the same p_c values would correspond to $g_c = 0.004$, or 0.4%. Adding another involuntary TES—or splitting an existing one into two—would alter the p_c values by only 4%, a trivial change. The p_c values selected thus fit all the criteria, insofar as it is possible to quantify the criteria. However, the criteria have wide enough limits to allow for the selection of other equally good p_c values and so to define the LOAs quantitatively and to set valid goals for risk reduction.

Although the device of using F at its current value is a useful one in establishing a set of p_c values, future upward variations in F, should these occur, are not a signal to raise the p_c values; rather, g_c would drop while the p_c values would remain the same—unless other factors showed they could be lowered. In this latter case, there is a parallel with setting lower safety incidence rate targets from time to time so as to improve overall safety performance.

V. THE THREE RISK REGIONS

Figure 1 summarizes graphically the risk regions, the relationships of the LOA and LOI, and their relationship to meeting the goal for cancer risk reduction. Figure 1 depicts these relationships for SESs of a single TES.

The LOA, essentially an individual or personal risk, is constant for a TES regardless of how many people (N) might be affected in any SES. The LOI, a group risk, is a function of the number of people in each SES as well as of other factors already discussed. For this reason the individual LOIs are depicted as short horizontal lines scattered above and below the dashed LOI trend line. So, when one SES is under scrutiny (see the plane outlined by straight, dashed lines), the LOA is that of the TES while the LOI is specific to that SES as shown. Exposure is symbolized by D in this figure.

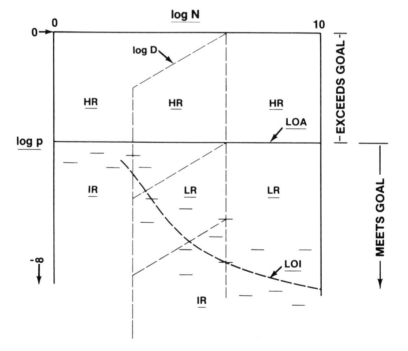

Figure 1   Risk regions.

For small enough N, and especially where background cancer rates are high, an LOI could be calculated higher than the LOA. The figure does not show this because the LOA is, by definition, a risk ceiling. For small groups, such as workers in a single work area, an arbitrarily defined LOI, for example, one tenth of the LOA, can be used to provide a gap or LR region between the LOA and the LOI.

There is a certain ethical value in the ceiling risk concept. When the goal is fully reached, individuals in different SESs may, on average, be at different levels of risk. However, at that juncture none, in pursuing their normal daily affairs and barring accident, will be exposed to average risks above the LOA. There is, of course, no way at the present time to account for especially sensitive individuals if such exist.

VI. APPLICATION OF THE RISK REGIONS

In taking the results of the second risk assessment stage, hazard evaluation, and combining them with the exposure distributions by types and routes developed during the exposure assessment to reach an ultimate conclusion as to the level of risk, it is soon discovered that the ranges within which human risk might lie are very broad.

A. An Example of a Risk Assessment

The first major use—and test—of this methodology, several years ago, was in the case of ethylene oxide. Animal data found a primary basis for the assessment, and therefore high-to-low-dosage extrapolation as well as interspecies extrapolation was required. Several of the commonly used fitting functions [12, 23] were found to fit the data well in the experimental range, but on extrapolation, as is often the case, they diverged widely from each other. Since there is no basis for believing that any of these functions represent the actual effects of ethylene oxide at low doses, such extrapolations can only be taken as possibilities in considering risks. All well-fitting extrapolations must therefore be included in a risk assessment.

In addition to the divergence of the various functions, other factors, when applied, add to the uncertainty of estimating risks at low doses. Dosing rate conversion from small laboratory animals to human-sized animals (the well-known "70 kg rat") are usually done several ways: on the mg/kg body weight basis, the mg/m² basis, and the ppm or concentration basis. Different results are obtained, which increases the range of responses predicted.

The prediction of actual, human risk from this nonexistent human-sized animal is usually not done except by assumption, though where ancillary information is available it may be possible to say, at least qualitatively, whether true human risk might be above or below such results. The usual assumption is that of equal sensitivity of species, though recent work indicates this may, on average, be a conservative assumption [24].

In addition to the aforementioned sources of uncertainty, the prediction of lifetime risk, when exposures are of various durations, and the stating of actual exposures, which are variable, in terms of the controlled doses administered to animals under test both add further uncertainties. Such transformations require pharmacokinetic information and information on the reduction of risk after cessation of dosing, neither of which is usually available. Here, too, assumptions usually need to be made, based on careful scientific judgment. The important thing is to display all of the extrapolations and all of the assumptions, demonstrating, where possible, the sensitivity of the results to variations in key assumptions.

Figure 2 shows a typical display of risk extrapolations against a background of the three risk regions. This display is typical of the many displays examined during the ethylene oxide risk assessment, each at fixed total duration of exposure. The lines marked A and B are the upper and lower bounds, respectively, of the region within which all the extrapolations lie, each corrected for dosing rate using more than one method. The dashed lines A' and B' illustrate the loci of the confidence limits corresponding to lines A and B. Clearly, the risk is depicted as lying within a wide band which widens further as dose (or exposure) decreases.

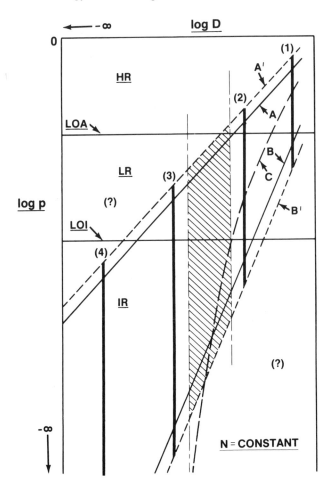

Figure 2   Using the risk regions to characterize risk.

In addition to the degree of uncertainty depicted in Figure 2, there is the fact that there is no known reason why the true, extrapolated risk must lie within the boundaries indicated. Curve C, for example, might be the true dose-response function, exhibiting what amounts to a threshold of effect, which is not unheard of for carcinogens [25, 26]. The two question marks in the figure indicate the further uncertainty as to where the true risk to humans might lie despite this broad approach to the utilization of animal data. One thing becomes clear after examining displays of this type: the less the extrapolation, the better in achieving even a modicum of certainty that a given level of risk exists. Thus, identifying a higher risk (HR) is less uncertain than identifying a lower risk (LR), and the identification of an insignificant risk is the least certain situation.

The four, numbered, vertical, heavy lines in Figure 2 indicate the range of risks that might exist at the corresponding dose levels. Line (1) would easily be judged as indicating a risk lying in the HR region, while line (4) would be judged to be in the IR region. Lines (2) and (3) pose some questions. Taking line (2) to denote a risk in the LR region is valid, despite some possibility the true risk might be in the HR region. The reason for this is that when a risk is characterized as lying in the LR region, reasonable steps are still taken to reduce the risk since the goal is as expressed by line (3). Thus, while work goes forward to improve the risk assessment, the risk is being reduced.

Line (3) probably indicates an insignificant risk though it lies partly in the LR region; in this case it would be wise to act to reduce risk as though it lay in the LR region. Since there is little reason to believe the risk lies in the HR region—other than the general uncertainty of this entire process—there would be little reason on the face of it to pursue significant work to improve the risk assessment. The experts required for this would be better employed in dealing with other, higher risks.

In actuality, exposures are found to cover a range of equivalent dosing rates, D, and to include a number of uncertainties and assumptions. This is indicated in Figure 2 by the cross-hatched area. This fact needs to be recognized; that it exists will not affect the general logic so far followed in deciding whether a risk lies in the HR, LR, or IR region.

B. Risk Response

Having concluded in which region the risk lies, the final question of what to do is resolved in the *risk response* stage. If it has been possible to carry out a quantitative risk assessment and a risk is found to lie in the HR region, action must be taken to reduce the risk so as to remove it from that region. This is in keeping with the goal for cancer reduction. Such actions may have to be taken in more than one step, following a carefully laid out, monitored plan.

If the risk is thought to lie in the LR region, reasonable actions to reduce the risk further should be taken, in keeping with the goal. If, however, the risk is thought to be insignificant, no action is warranted since the level of risk cannot be observed and may even be zero; monitoring and control are needed in this case, as in the others, to ensure that the risk remains insignificant.

Much space has been devoted to quantification, but for reasons already given, this is not to signify that qualitative risk assessment is not useful. In the case of qualitative risk assessment, it may only be possible to conclude that a risk requiring reduction exists. Here the risk would be treated as lying in the LR region and steps would be taken, accordingly, to reduce the risk while conducting the work needed to better characterize the risk.

VII. CONCLUSIONS

In certain respects the methodology described has generic characteristics. Experience shows that individual carcinogens behave so differently, one from the another in the same species as well as between species, that a simple generic scheme of broad and easy application is a practical and scientific impossibility. Given that a thorough scientific and technical study is required for each carcinogen and its exposure circumstances, there is nevertheless one characteristic, risk, which links separate carcinogens. Once determined, the level of risk indicates the general priority, urgency and intensity with which the risk is to be reduced—though specific actions must be tailored to specific circumstances of exposure. The stagewise process of risk assessment and response, together with the pragmatically defined risk regions, provide the mechanism and support for carrying out what might be considered the generic aspects of this methodology.

The methodology has so far found application only in workplace situations though the derivation of the p_c values involves a consideration of all TESs. This situation is likely to persist since, as a practical matter, a private firm has the ability to deal most easily and directly with the workplace, where necessary, beyond the requirements of regulatory compliance. There is an impact of all independent risk-reducing activity, however, that goes beyond a particular firm's workplace. This "ripple effect" comes from the fact that when a risk is reduced, the common practice is not only to inform workers but also to inform customers. Thus, workers (and customers) beyond those of a firm which has acted to reduce risk can also benefit by these activities.

A major problem with human risk assessment, quantitative or qualitative, using this methodology or another is the slimness of its foundations and the shakiness of its structure. This must be kept in mind when considering risk response alternatives. Nonetheless, members of a risk assessment group, following a logical sequence in assessing risks and in determining the ultimate risk level, are caused to communicate their knowledge to each other and to think deeply as they reach their conclusions in the face of high uncertainty. There is a distinct advantage, too, in being able to justify, and therefore to pursue, the risk reduction recommendations that emerge through the use of a systematic approach. Looking to the future, as the scientific basis for interpreting dose-time-response data at low doses and in human terms is improved, the methodology described here will become all the more easily applied.

REFERENCES

1. J. Higginson and C. S. Muir, Environmental carcinogenesis: Misconceptions and limitations to cancer control, *J. Natl. Cancer Inst., 63*:1291–1298 (1979).
2. R. Doll and R. Peto, *The Causes of Cancer*, Oxford University Press, Oxford (1981).
3. Occupational Safety and Health Administration (OSHA), Occupational exposure to ethylene oxide, *Fed. Reg., 48*:17,284–17,319 (1983).
4. P. F. Deisler, Jr., Dealing with industrial health risks: A step-wise, goal-oriented concept, in *American Association for the Advancement of Science Special Symposium No. 65: Risk in a Technological Society*

(C. Hohenenser and J. X. Kasperson, eds.), Westview Press, Boulder, Colo. (1982).

5. P. F. Deisler, Jr., A goal-oriented approach to reducing industrially related carcinogenic risks, *Drug Metab. Rev.*, *13(5)*:875-911 (1982).

6. P. F. Deisler, Jr., J. E. Berger, and R. L. Brunner, A systematic approach to reducing the risk of industrially related cancer, *Reg. Toxicol. Pharmacol.*, *3*:26-27 (1983).

7. P. F. Deisler, Jr., Fundamental problems and practical solutions in assessing and abating risks that chronic chemical exposures pose for people, presented at the Meeting of the American Association for the Advancement of Science, Santa Barbara, California, June 23, 1982.

8. P. F. Deisler, Jr., Utilization of risk assessment in corporate risk management decisions, presented at the Chemical Manufacturers Association Symposium on Risk Management of Existing Chemicals, Washington, D.C., Dec. 8, 1983 (proceedings to be published).

9. P. F. Deisler, Jr., Impact of cancer in industry, presented at the Seminar on Cancer Prevention and Control sponsored by the Texas Department of Health and the Texas Chemical Council, inter alia, San Antonio, Texas, Jan. 27, 1984 (proceedings to be published).

10. D. R. Calkins, R. L. Dixon, C. R. Gerber, D. Zarin, and G. S. Omenn, Identification, characterization, and control of potential human carcinogens: A framework for federal decision-making, *J. Natl. Cancer Inst.*, *64(1)*:169-176 (1980).

11. P. F. Deisler, Jr., Science, regulations and the safe handling of chemicals, *Reg. Toxicol. Pharmacol.*, *2*:335-344 (1982).

12. Food Safety Council, *Proposed System for Food Safety Assessment*, Final Report of the Scientific Committee of the Food Safety Council, Wash., D.C., June, 1980. (See also *Fd. Cosmet. Toxicol.*, *18*:711-734 (1980).

13. ECETOC, *Risk Assessment of Occupational Chemical Carcinogens*, Monograph No. 3, European Chemical Industry Ecology and Toxicology Center (ECETOC), Brussels, Belgium, Jan. 1982.

14. National Research Council, *Risk Assessment in the Federal Government: Managing the Process*, National Academy Press, Washington, D.C., 1983.

15. Office of Technology Assessment (OTA), *Assessment of Technologies for Determining Cancer Risks from the Environment*, U.S. Government Printing Office, Washington, D.C., June 1981.

16. Food and Drug Administration (FDA), Chemical compounds in food-producing animals, *Fed. Reg.*, *44*:17,070 (1979).

17. T. C. Byerly, *USDA Policy on Carcinogens* (Contract 43-32R7-9-1100), July 2, 1979.

18. Environmental Protection Agency (EPA), Requests for comments on water quality criteria for 27 toxic water pollutants, *Fed. Reg., 44*: 15,926 (1979).
19. United States Supreme Court, *Industrial Union Department, AFL-CIO v. American Petroleum Institute, et al.*, No. 78-911, decided July 2, 1980.
20. C. Starr, *Perspectives on Benefit-Risk Decision Making*, National Academy of Engineering, 1972.
21. R. Wilson, Direct testimony before the United States Department of Labor Assistant Secretary of Labor for Occupational Safety and Health Administration, OSHA Docket No. H-090, Washington, D.C., 1978.
22. J. G. Cobler and F. D. Hoerger, Analysis of agency estimates of risk for carcinogenic agents, in *Proceedings of the Symposium on Risk Analysis in the Private Sector*, Third Annual Meeting of the Society for Risk Analysis, New York, 1983 (V. T. Covello and C. Whipple, eds.), Plenum Press, New York (in press).
23. C. N. Park and R. D. Snee, Quantitative risk assessment: State-of-the-art for carcinogenesis, *Fund. Appl. Toxicol., 3*:320-333 (1983).
24. R. H. Adamson and S. M. Sieber, Chemical carcinogenesis studies in nonhuman primates, in *Organ and Species Specificity in Chemical Carcinogenesis*, (R. Langenbach, S. Nesnow and J. M. Rice, eds.), Plenum Press, New York, 1983.
25. T. Y. Chin, R. W. Tyl, J. A. Popp, and H. d'A. Heck, Chemical urolithiasis 1. Characteristics of bladder stone induction by terephthalic acid and dimethyl terephthalate in weaning Fischer-344 rats, *Toxicol. Appl. Pharmacol., 58*:307-321 (1981).
26. R. L. Anderson, C. L. Alden, and J. A. Merski, The effects of nitrilotriacetate on cation disposition and urinary tract toxicity, *Food Chem. Toxicol., 20(1)*:105-122 (Feb. 1982).

8

CANCER CONTROL IN THE WORKPLACE: SOME EXAMPLES FROM THE UTILITY INDUSTRY

Leonard A. Sagan and Chris G. Whipple
Electric Power Research Institute
Palo Alto, California

I. INTRODUCTION

Bringing electricity to residential and business customers requires three basic processes: the generation of electric power at a generating station; the transmission of that electrical energy from the generating site to substations, since transmission voltages are generally too high to be used directly; and the distribution of electricity to customers. At the substation, the voltage is stepped down through the use of transformers to voltages appropriate for consumer use. These lower voltages are transmitted over distribution systems.

Approximately 3300 utility systems are involved in generation, transmission, distribution, or all three. The major energy sources for electricity production are coal, oil, gas, uranium, and hydroelectric power.

The electric utility industry is one of the nation's largest employers, with more than 500,000 persons employed. Capital investment exceeds 200 billion dollars, and industry revenues were roughly 120 billion dollars in 1982. Ownership of the industry is divided between the private sector, which operates many of the largest companies, and several thousand mostly smaller companies. These latter are operated by governmental bodies such as municipalities, are run by cooperative associations, or are directed by federal entities such as the huge Tennessee Valley Authority or Bonneville Power Association. Most of the municipal power companies buy energy from the private companies or federal agencies and distribute it to their customers.

The utility industry has some interesting attributes from the perspective of occupational health. Since electric utilities operate throughout the 50 states, there is enormous geographic variability. Also, since much utility equipment is necessarily outdoors and requires maintenance throughout the year, personnel are exposed to severe extremes of climate and working conditions, varying from the heat of the desert in the Southwest to the frigid winters of the north. Many utilities are also engaged in a variety of other activities, ranging from the operation of coal and uranium mines, railroad systems, and construction teams to research laboratories.

Medical programs among utilities vary enormously: smaller companies typically have no full-time medical personnel, but have contractual arrangements with local physicians and hospitals. Larger utilities may have fairly extensive medical staffs, nursing stations, and highly developed preventive health examination programs. The same is true of industrial hygiene services: there is a wide spectrum of arrangements for the use and utilization of hygienists. No industry-wide study of cancer incidence is known to exist.

What has been said of clinical resources is also true of research activities. Some utilities or groups of utilities may engage in ad hoc research efforts. One example, ESEERCO, a consortium of New York utilities, has undertaken research directed to the issue of a possible relationship between electromagnetic fields and cancer.

Also providing research support for its member utilities is the Electric Power Research Institute (EPRI) in Palo Alto, California. Within its Environmental Assessment Department, EPRI maintains an occupational health research effort which includes a component directed to research in cancer. One current EPRI project involves the taking of an inventory of chemicals found within the utility workplace with the intention of ranking these in some order of hazard. Hazard will be determined on the basis of the numbers of persons exposed, the magnitude of the exposure, and the toxicity of the chemical.

The industry also coordinates its responses to regulatory and legislative initiatives through its trade associations; for example, when questions arose as to the safety of polychlorinated biphenyls (PCBs), a substance which had always been assumed to be safe, the industry was quickly able to bring resources to bear on the issue of the scientific merit of PCB toxicity and to quickly mobilize its safety efforts.

In comparison, for example, with the synthetic chemical industry, there are few known carcinogenic agents with which the utility industry deals regularly. In this brief report, we will illustrate industry practices by selecting five very different agents for discussion: ionizing radiation, nonionizing radiation, asbestos, polychlorinated biphenyls, and inorganic arsenic. Three of these, inorganic arsenic, asbestos, and ionizing radiation are well recognized carcinogens at high exposure levels but have not been shown to be carcinogenic at levels at which they are found in the utility industry. In the case of PCBs and nonionizing radiation, hazard to human populations has not been demonstrated; however, because of public speculation about these agents, some discussion will be devoted to them. The last to be discussed, though briefly, is nonionizing radiation. It has not been considered a hazard to human populations, but is mentioned to illustrate how the industry maintains its awareness of scientific reports in fields of possible interest.

II. IONIZING RADIATION

There are now approximately eighty nuclear reactors generating electricity in the United States. The number of sites is considerably less since two or more reactors are frequently located at the same site and share personnel.

There are approximately 50,000 utility personnel engaged in the operation of these reactor facilities. In addition, contract personnel who may be required to assist in fueling and other maintenance operations must also be trained and monitored by the utility. This staff will grow considerably in numbers as new reactors are completed and begin operation. The plants now under construction will roughly double the nuclear generating capacity of the industry over the next several years.

The construction, licensing, and operation of these facilities are all regulated by the U.S. Nuclear Regulatory Commission (NRC). In addition, each state maintains a radiation protection agency which is also responsible for surveillance and control of radiation exposures.

A. General Risk Considerations

Occupational exposures to nuclear plant personnel are due to both fission products (i.e., the byproducts of the fission of reactor fuel) and activation products produced when materials are exposed to high levels of radiation. The most basic level of occupational protection is provided by radiation shielding where necessary, but exposure nevertheless occurs because some contamination of the reactor coolant results from the diffusion or leakage of fission products from reactor fuel. Exposure is largely due to maintenance and refueling activities. The level of exposure within the reactor building tends to increase slowly with plant age, as the quantity of activation products increases, but the amount of exposure varies greatly depending on design differences, maintenance practices, and other factors.

With the possible exception of cigarette smoking, the cancer risk from exposure to ionizing radiation is better known than that from any other carcinogenic agent. Radiation risk factors are particularly well known at high doses, principally as a result of extensive studies of atomic bomb survivors and of persons who have been occupationally or therapeutically exposed. The extensive studies [1] of watch dial painters exposed to radium and also of patients treated for rheumatoid spondylitis by radiation both provide information regarding human risks from radiation.

The accumulated epidemiologic data, as well as the extensive experimental animal literature, are regularly reviewed by a number of radiation protection agencies, including the U.S. National Academy of Sciences BEIR Committee (Biological Effects of Ionizing Radiation) [2]. Although populations of persons exposed at occupational levels do not exist in sufficient numbers to validate risk factors derived from higher doses, the conservative assumption has been made that the risks at low doses are linear or proportional to those effects seen at higher doses. With the possible exception of cancer, no significant health effects would be expected from occupational radiation exposures, based on the experience of other exposed human populations.

Guided by these generally accepted assumptions, the standards generated by the radiation protection community and promulgated by the NRC permit annual exposures to an individual averaging no more than 5 rem. In actual experience, the average worker in the nuclear industry receives an annual exposure of 0.8 rem, and of all exposed persons less than 1% receive as much as

5 rem. Current estimates based on the generally accepted assumptions are that for each 10,000 person-rems of radiation exposure, one to two fatal cancers may eventually occur. For example, if 10,000 persons were each exposed to 1 rem, then the aggregate exposure would be 10,000 person-rem, from which one or two cancer cases would be expected. Such a population would normally be expected to experience approximately 1600 fatal cancers as a result of other and largely unknown causes, so the total would then be 1601–1602 cases. Use of this risk factor indicates that current annual exposures increase cancer risk to the average exposed workers by roughly one chance in 10,000 over their lifetimes; this amount of risk is considerably less than that due to the exposure variation experienced among the geographic regions of the United States. Since such a small increase cannot be detected in human populations because of the variability among populations, this excess has never been substantiated and may, in fact, be zero. Because the risk estimate cited is based on the assumption that effects at low doses are proportional to those at high doses where repair mechanisms cannot operate, the risk estimate is viewed by many as likely to be an overestimate. For example, the National Academy of Sciences most recent report [2] suggests that a linear-quadratic dose-response function, a formulation which would produce a lower risk at low doses, would be more appropriate.

B. Safety Management Methods

Many of the safety management methods adopted for ionizing radiation are similar to those used for other agents which are known to be carcinogenic at high exposure levels. Those techniques include: training, monitoring of exposures, research, and medical screening.

Training is required of all monitored personnel, both when first employed as well as on a periodic basis thereafter. The content of training courses is specified by the NRC. The training specifies the use of protective devices and procedures as well as basic knowledge of radiation protection and risk. The trainers are generally utility employees. A loose organization of radiation trainers has recently been formed to share experiences and improve training materials.

Every reactor operator is required to provide an adequate staff of trained health physicists to monitor procedures and exposures. Exposure records for the company must be submitted to the NRC on an annual basis or, for individual employees, at the time of termination. Monitoring consists of area monitoring, personnel dosimetry, and whole body counting on an annual or more frequent basis. This latter technique provides assurance that there has been no inhalation or ingestion of radioactive materials.

Several of the larger U.S. utilities have initiated on-going epidemiological studies of their exposed employees. This research is prospective in nature and will produce results at a future time. Ontario Hydro has analyzed mortality data of its employees since 1970 and has recently reported that cancer deaths and leukemia appear unrelated to radiation doses. In this study, actual cases have been below the statistical expectations [3]. British Nuclear Fuels Limited also has made a long-term study with similar results.

Medical surveillance is also required by all utilities. Utility practices are likely to differ, depending upon company policy and job requirements. For example, reactor operators are required to have psychological as well as conventional medical examinations.

C. Nuclear Plant Safety

Almost certainly the greatest investments in the management of carcinogenic risks by the utility industry are for the avoidance of nuclear power plant accidents. The basic approach to public protection is the use of multiple barriers between the fission products and the external environment. This "defense in depth" approach, as it is known, provides four levels of containment: the uranium fuel (and subsequently the mixture of fission products) is embedded in ceramic elements with an extremely high melting point; elements are loaded into zirconium alloy tubes to make fuel rods; bundles of fuel rods are kept within a primary system (i.e., reactor pressure vessel and piping); and the primary system is surrounded by a thick reinforced concrete containment building.

Extensive use is made of conservative engineering criteria and redundant safety systems and, in addition, plant sites are typically far from population centers with a required exclusion area surrounding each plant.

In the mid-1970s, the first attempt was made to perform an assessment of public risks from nuclear power plants. The Reactor Safety Study [4] used systems analysis techniques to try to identify the most important accident sequences and to quantitatively describe the public risks arising from these accident sequences. The estimated effects were quite small; for example, the expectation value (which may not capture the public interpretation of low probability-high consequence risks) was about 0.02 latent cancer fatalities per reactor year. Other effects such as early fatalities and illness and thyroid nodules were considered and were also estimated to pose quite small risks. These results were controversial, given the widespread debate that was then going on regarding nuclear reactor safety. At that time, most attention was focused on the overall risk estimates rather than on the engineering insights that were developed in the analysis. It was also assumed at the time that the results of the Reactor Safety Study (of one boiling water reactor and one pressurized water reactor) were representative of nuclear power plants in general.

Since 1975, roughly 20 additional probabilistic risk assessments of nuclear power plants have been conducted, and the levels of detail and sophistication of the approach have increased substantially. The application of such studies has also changed. It is now conventional wisdom among reactor safety analysts that their value lies not in the overall risk estimate (the Director of Risk Analysis at the NRC refers to this preoccupation as "terminal bottom line disease"), but rather with what is revealed regarding the contribution of various plant systems and failure modes to public risk. Taken as a body, these studies have led to changes in emphasis in safety research and analysis, and to a belief among nuclear safety analysts that power plant risks are sensitive to individual plant characteristics rather than to the basic design concept. These studies have also highlighted the significance of external risks such as earthquakes, and the performance of plant operators and maintenance people.

As the use of probabilistic analyses has grown in the industry, so too have the incentives to use such analyses for regulatory purposes. Coincidentally, in response to recommendations of the President's Commission on the Accident at Three Mile Island, the NRC committed to try to develop "an explicit policy statement on safety philosophy and the role of safety-cost tradeoffs in the NRC safety decisions" [5]. Thus the NRC began in 1980 to attempt to develop explicit safety goals for commercial nuclear power plants. After holding a number of workshops and considering a number of suggestions, the NRC issued a proposed policy statement for comment which explicitly defined safety criteria and the underlying philosophical rationale for public protection. The NRC has since established a two-year evaluation period during which an implementation plan will be developed.

The proposed safety guides [5] consist of two qualitative goals and several quantitative design objectives. The qualitative goals are: first, that individual members of the public should be provided a level of protection from the consequences of nuclear power plant operation such that individuals bear no significant additional risk to life and health, and second, that societal risks to life and health from nuclear power plant operation should be comparable to or less than the risks of generating electricity by viable competing technologies and should not be a significant addition to other societal risks.

The quantitative design objectives consist of three parts. The first part deals with individual and societal mortality risks: the risk to an average individual in the vicinity of a nuclear power plant of prompt fatalities that might result from reactor accidents should not exceed one-tenth of one percent (0.1%) of the sum of prompt fatality risks resulting from other accidents to which members of the U.S. population are generally exposed; moreover, the risk to the population in the area near a nuclear power plant of cancer fatalities that might result from nuclear power plant operation should not exceed one-tenth of one percent (0.1%) of the sum of cancer fatality risks resulting from all other causes.

The second part is a benefit-cost guideline: the benefit of an incremental reduction of societal mortality risks should be compared with the associated costs on the basis of $1000 per person-rem averted. Finally, the third part is a plant performance design objective: the likelihood of a nuclear reactor accident that results in a large-scale core melt should normally be less than one in 10,000 per year of reactor operation.

In proposing these safety goals, the NRC made a comment relevant to the difficulty of safety decisions which are viewed differently in hindsight than in prospect:

> We want to make clear that no death attributable to nuclear power plant operation will ever be "acceptable" in the sense that the Commission would regard it as a routine or permissible event. We are discussing acceptable risks, not acceptable deaths. In any fatal accident, a course of conduct posing an acceptable risk at one moment results in an unacceptable death moments later. This is true whether one speaks of driving, swimming, flying, or generating electricity from coal. Each of these activities poses a calculable risk to society and to individuals. Some of those who accept the risk (or are part of a society that accepts risk) do not survive it. We intend that no such accident(s) will occur, but the possibility cannot be entirely eliminated. Furthermore, individual and societal risks are less than the risk that society is now exposed to from each of the other activities mentioned above.

III. NONIONIZING RADIATION

This radiation does not produce ionization in materials or in tissues, and is not known to have biologic effects other than sensory perception of high field strengths, felt as a tingling of the skin. Several recent studies, however, have suggested that persons engaging in occupations exposed to high electromagnetic fields are at increased risk of cancer [6, 7]. These results are in some dispute. For example, no measurements were available to support the assumption of increased exposure, and other investigators have failed to find such a relationship [8]. A full literature review is in preparation [9].

In order to evaluate these reports, EPRI and several utilities have undertaken measurements of exposure levels for both occupational personnel as well as members of the public. At present, electric field exposures are not generally considered to pose a risk of cancer.

IV. POLYCHLORINATED BIPHENYLS (PCBs)

Polychlorinated biphenyls (PCBs) have been purchased and used in the utility industry for decades in dielectric fluids for transformers and capacitors. Their wide use results from the fact that they are highly fire resistant and otherwise have electrical properties nearly as good as those of mineral oil. Since PCBs are somewhat more expensive than mineral oil, they are generally found in use only where transformers are in buildings or in other locations where fire-retardant qualities are important. Of the 20 million transformers in use today in the utility industry, about 20,000 are filled with PCBs. The almost 3,000,000 capacitors (devices which control voltages on transmission and distribution lines) contain PCBs. PCBs are the only substances specifically mandated in the Toxic Substances Control Act, Section 6(e) for regulatory control by the Environmental Protection Agency.

Exposures to PCBs occur because transformers and capacitors must be regularly inspected and repaired. The electrical properties of the fluid may change with time and therefore must be regularly tested. Furthermore, transformers may deteriorate, develop leaks, accumulate debris, and require cleaning.

Some controversy and considerable uncertainty exists with respect to the long-term toxic properties of PCBs. The toxicology of these materials is complex and cannot be reviewed here. Briefly, while studies have demonstrated that PCBs are liver carcinogens in some animal species, there are inconsistencies in the data which make interpretation difficult. Polychlorinated biphenyls are chlorinated aromatic hydrocarbons. Since the degree of chlorination and the position of the chlorine atoms may vary, PCBs actually are a large class of compounds whose toxic properties are not identical.

The human data which do exist have been interpreted by some as explainable on the basis of contaminants such as chlorinated dibenzofurans and dioxins which can appear in used PCBs. In the largest known human exposure, that which occurred in an unfortunate accident in Japan in which cooking oil was contaminated with PCBs, a variety of serious but transient health effects observed have been attributed to the relatively high levels of contaminants found in the oil as a result of being heated to high temperatures during the cooking process [10]. These contaminants would not be expected to be present in electric utility equipment under usual conditions, nor would utility employees be likely to ingest PCBs. At this time, neither the exposed Japanese population nor any of the occupationally exposed populations have been found to exhibit an elevated risk of cancer [11]. Liver enzyme changes and hepatomegaly have been observed, however, among heavily exposed persons.

NIOSH has estimated that some 100,000 electrical workers in the United States are potentially exposed to PCBs. One report of federal employees who are engaged in the maintenance of transformers indicates that 79% worked in areas which exceeded OSHA standards for permissible air concentrations [12]. On the other hand, in a limited study of two utilities, one private and one public, NIOSH found air concentrations of PCBs to be well below those specified by the OSHA standards. Serum levels among employees in these same facilities were inexplicably lower for those exposed to PCBs than for those who were not, and considerably lower than for those employed in a transformer manufacturing plant [13].

Protection of personnel working with PCBs requires, above all, good judgment, planning, and training. When exposures are anticipated, disposable protective clothing is worn. This includes coveralls, plastic overshoes, gloves, and face shields. Normally, respiratory equipment is not required because of the low vapor pressure of PCBs. However, if the employee enters an enclosed space where PCBs have been spilled, and if the space has not been ventilated, then respiratory equipment is normally required. If the skin is accidentally exposed, thorough washing with soap and water is adequate. If there has been an exceptional exposure, then the attending physician may wish to obtain a serum sample in order to determine the degree of absorption.

V. INORGANIC ARSENIC

The carcinogenicity of inhaled or ingested inorganic arsenic to both the skin and the lung of humans has been demonstrated under certain circumstances of exposure. Much of the data for lung cancer comes from studies of smelter workers [14], and the current OSHA standard ($10 \mu g/m^3$) is based on this information. There exist a number of factors of uncertainty regarding this data, however. One of these uncertainties regards the shape of the dose-response relationship, and this in turn results from the poor quality of the exposure data. Secondly, the effect of cigarette smoking as a factor in arsenic carcinogenesis is not clear. Furthermore, since fumes from smeltering processes produce complex mixtures containing a number of other metals as well as gases, the interactions which may occur among these substances and inorganic arsenic need to be clarified. Carcinogenicity has not been demonstrated in animal studies, but toxicologically, selenium and arsenic are antagonistic. There is also knowledge that the two oxidation states of arsenic, the trivalent and the pentavalent state, differ in their toxicity to animals. Whether or not the two valence states differ in their carcinogenicity is an unsettled matter.

Exposure to arsenic in the utility industry arises from two quite different sources, geothermal energy production and exposure to hopper and precipitator ash.

In geothermal energy production, the steam source itself contains a very low concentration of arsenic. The single situation where protective measures must be taken is in the cleaning of turbine blades which have become encrusted with arsenic salts. Such operations are carried out by a relatively few persons on infrequent occasions. Respiratory equipment and protective clothing are required and provide adequate protection.

The second potential situation in which arsenic exposures are a theoretical threat occurs because respirable fly ash particles tend to collect arsenic on their surfaces as the particles cool and combustion gases condense. Whether this arsenic can be eluted from such particles by biological fluids following ingestion or inhalation is currently the subject of an EPRI project.

VI. ASBESTOS

Over the past 25 years, evidence that exposure to asbestos produces a variety of diseases of the lungs, including asbestosis, mesothelioma, and lung cancer, has been accumulated. This evidence has been gathered from epidemiologic studies of a variety of industries. In some of these studies demonstrating increased risk, the industrial exposure was relatively short, lasting only a few years, but most studies indicate latent periods as long as 20 years or even longer. In instances in which the exposures were intense, as much as 20% of workers have developed asbestos-related diseases. It has also been demonstrated that there is a strong interaction with cigarette smoking [15], as shown in Table 1.

Because of the excellent thermal insulating properties of asbestos, it has been extensively used in electrical generating stations to insulate piping. Although the manufacture and use of asbestos for this purpose has been prohibited since 1973, repairs of older plants continue to create potential exposure conditions to utility employees.

OSHA regulations now require the use of wetting agents to reduce dust concentrations, respiratory equipment, and annual medical examinations.

Table 1 Relative Risks of Lung Cancer According to Exposure to Asbestos and to Cigarette Smoking [15]

Asbestos exposure	Cigarette smoking	
	No	Yes
No	1.0	10.9
Yes	5.2	53.2

Although no data exist on the extent or magnitude of exposures under these circumstances, such "rip out" work may create high exposure conditions if no care is taken to reduce exposures. For example, one study of such work demonstrated air concentrations of a few hundred fibers per cubic centimeter, whereas the threshold limit value is two fibers per cubic centimeter [16]. OSHA has recently issued a new emergency temporary standard for asbestos [17] of 0.5 fibers per cubic centimeter and a new, permanent rule making is in the offing at this writing (December 1983).

VII. SUMMARY

The electric utility industry is a large and diverse industry where the majority of employees are not exposed to significant quantities of carcinogenic materials. As indicated by the examples offered above, the approach adopted for each agent is tailored to the particular needs dictated by usage and available knowledge. With well understood or historically significant risks such as ionizing radiation and asbestos, the emphasis is on training and compliance with regulations and other established procedures, coupled with a carefully documented program of monitoring. Current research is directed to collecting exposure data and health statistics. For newer and less well characterized hazards such as PCBs, the emphasis is on limiting exposures and complying with existing regulations. For highly speculative issues such as nonionizing radiation, the industry emphasis is necessarily on research.

REFERENCES

1. J. Boice and C. Land, *Ionizing Radiation in Cancer Epidemiology and Prevention*, (D. Schottenfeld and J. Fraumeni, eds.), W. B. Saunders Co., Philadelphia, 1982.
2. National Academy of Sciences/National Research Council Committee on the Biological Effects of Ionizing Radiation, *The Effects of Exposure to Low Levels of Ionizing Radiation*, Washington, D.C., 1980.
3. *Nucleonics Week*, p. 6. (October 20, 1983).
4. U.S. Nuclear Regulatory Commission, *Reactor Safety Study: An Assess-*

ment of Accident Risks in U.S. Commercial Nuclear Power Plants, WASH-1400, October 1975.

5. U.S. Nuclear Regulatory Commission, *Safety Goals for Nuclear Power Plants: A Discussion Paper*, NUREG-OBBO for Comment, February 1982; also NUREG-DBBO Revision L, *Safety Goals for Nuclear Power Plant Operation*, May 1973.

6. N. Wertheimer and E. Leeper, Electrical wiring configurations and cancer, *Am. J. Epidemiol., 109*:173-183 (1979).

7. S. Milham, Mortality from leukemia in workers exposed to electrical and magnetic fields, *N. Engl. J. Med., 307*:249 (1982).

8. J. Fulbon, P. Cobb, et al., Electrical wiring configurations and childhood leukemia in Rhode Island, *Am. J. Epidemiol. 111*:292-296 (1980).

9. M. G. Morgan, D. R. Lincoln, I. Nair, and H. K. Florig, An exploration of risk assessment needs and opportunities for possible health consequences from *50/60 HZ Electromagnetic Fields*, Dept. of Engineering and Public Policy, Carnegie-Mellon University (in preparation).

10. M. Kuratsune, Epidemiologic studies on Yusho, in *PCB Poisoning and Pollution*, (K. Higuchi, ed.) Academic Press, New York, 1976.

11. D. Brown and M. Jones, Mortality and industrial hygiene study of workers exposed to polychlorinated biphenyls, *Arch. Environmental Health, 36*:120-129 (1981).

12. C. L. Moseley, C. Geraci, and J. Burg, Polychlorinated biphenyl exposure in transformer maintenance operations, *Am. Ind. Hyg. Assoc. J. 43*:170-174 (1983).

13. A. Smith, J. Schloemer, et al., Metabolic and health consequences of occupational exposure to polychlorinated biphenyls, *Br. J. Ind. Med., 39*:361-369 (1982).

14. W. Lederer and R. Fensterheim, *Arsenic: Industrial, Biomedical, Environmental Perspectives*, Van Nostrand, New York, 1983.

15. E. Hammond, I. Selikoff, and H. Seidman, Asbestos, cigarette smoking, and death rates, *Ann. N.Y. Acad. Sci., 330*:473-490 (1979).

16. W. Reitze, Application of sprayed inorganic fiber containing asbestos: Occupational occupational health hazards, *Am. Ind. Hyg. Assoc. J., 33*:178-191 (1972).

17. OSHA Emergency Temporary Standard, *Fed. Reg., 48*:51086-51140 (November 4, 1983).

9

THE HISTORY AND ACCOMPLISHMENTS OF THE OCCUPATIONAL SAFETY AND HEALTH ADMINISTRATION IN REDUCING CANCER RISKS

Jacqueline K. Corn and Morton Corn*
Department of Environmental Health Sciences
The Johns Hopkins University
School of Hygiene and Public Health
Baltimore, Maryland

---

*Formerly Assistant Secretary of Labor for Occupational Safety and Health, Washington, D.C.

I. INTRODUCTION

A. Different National Regulatory Philosophies with Regard to Carcinogens

A net of federal regulations promulgated in the United States to deal with the increased production of potentially toxic chemicals has been documented elsewhere [1]. These initiatives were a response to the early perception of the presence of chemicals in commercial usage in the United States which, as of 1978, were reported to number about 63,000 [2]. The decision by the United States government to protect public health and the environment from chemical hazards was not unique. Other nations also approached regulation of chemicals in the environment (see Chapter 10). Comparable regulations have been passed in France, Britain, West Germany, and Sweden [3].

Although all of these regulatory initiatives occurred during the post-World War II period when concepts of risk and safety were not well defined, their passage was predicated on an implicit, unarticulated concept of risk and risk assessment. Lowrance introduced the idea that safety is a relative term which designates an acceptable level of risk by an individual, a group, or society in general [4]. The Committee on Risk Assessment further elaborated on these concepts to define the scientific process of calculating the probability of occurrence of an untoward event as "risk assessment," and the sociotechnical process of arriving at an acceptable level of societal risk as "risk management" [5]. Risk assessment procedures incorporate scientific assumptions or "inference guidelines" into the analysis and result in the generation of a mathematical probability, with confidence limits, for the undesirable event occurring. This is a form of quantitative risk assessment. In the next ten years we shall see increased efforts to further develop the science of risk assessment and the necessary procedures and inference guidelines may well be institutionalized by U.S. regulatory agencies.

Early on, cancer was a focus of the regulations for chemical control in westernized nations. Although fewer than 60 chemicals have been evaluated as cancer hazards to humans in epidemiological studies, and approximately 350 chemicals are suspect human carcinogens based upon studies in experimental animals and limited human observations [6], there has been a major U.S. regulatory effort to address carcinogens. The emphasis on carcinogens has been greater in the United States than elsewhere, perhaps stemming from 1958 with the enactment of the Delaney Amendment to the Federal Food, Drug and Cosmetic Act. Although the so-called Delaney Clause did not directly call for adoption of a national cancer policy, its presence has come to be construed as such by many sectors of the population. The Delaney Clause calls for banning of any deliberate food additive which is carcinogenic, as defined by appropriate animal testing or human experience. It is a relatively simple and straightforward rule. As time passed, it has been increasingly regarded as too simple for the regulation of chemical carcinogens. The earliest effort to address carcinogen regulation in a non-substance-by-substance manner through the use of a generic standard, was that by the Occupational Safety and Health Administration (OSHA) to develop generic regulations for the identification and classification of carcinogens [7]. Attempts by the Interagency Regulatory Liaison Group followed those of OSHA.

In many instances, the United States approaches chemical carcinogen regulation on the basis of permitting an "acceptable" risk. The lowest "feasible" or "practicable" exposure levels are the targets for regulation. U.S. statutes do not in general ban chemicals, though some permit banning as one alternative. OSHA, in particular, utilizes Permissible Exposure Limits (PEL) which, in the case of carcinogens, are the lowest limits that are feasibly achievable. For example, on November 2, 1983, OSHA issued an Emergency Temporary Standard for asbestos-in-air of 0.5 fibers/cc of air, averaged over an eight-hour working period [8]. OSHA also enforces a host of prescriptive, detailed work practices which accompany the requirement for the PEL in the asbestos standard. Other nations ban asbestos usage entirely. For example, Sweden, the Netherlands, Denmark and Norway essentially ban all forms of asbestos [9]. The regulatory decision to ban usage of a carcinogen can be phrased as a statement by a society to not accept any level of health risk associated with exposure to the substance.

B. Past Regulatory Priorities of OSHA as Reflected in Rulemaking

The Occupational Safety and Health Administration was permitted two years from promulgation of the Occupational Safety and Health Act (OSH Act) to adopt as legal standards, by agency administrative action, any health and safety standards in either preexisting federal laws or in guidelines adopted by consensus groups. OSHA adopted a large number of standards on this basis. Included in these standards were many of the 1968 threshold limit values (TLVs) for airborne agents of the American Conference of Governmental Industrial Hygienists (ACGIH) which were included in the Walsh-Healey Public Contracts Act list and which included some chemical carcinogens. Some of the standards adopted were those of the American National Standards Institute (ANSI); where these existed, they preempted the ACGIH standards (for example, benzene). After the two-year period referred to, OSHA had to undertake rulemaking, adhering to the U.S. Administrative Procedures Act of 1956, to establish permanent standards, as described later in this chapter. The proven or suspect chemical carcinogens covered by OSHA in its early adoption of existing TLVs are listed in Table 1. Those substances for which permanent standard rulemaking was later undertaken are so designated.

Because extensive agency resources must be committed to permanent standard rulemaking and the process is long and involved, the agency should carefully consider agents or practices for the subject of such rulemaking. Insight can be gained into OSHA past priorities by reviewing the permanent health standards promulgated by OSHA since it inception. OSHA operates under a

Table 1 List of Chemical Carcinogens Regulated by OSHA for Airborne Concentrations [6]

2-Acetylaminofluorene[a]	3,3-Dichlorbenzidine[a]
Acrylonitrile[a]	4-Dimethylaminoazobenzene[a]
4-Aminodiphenyl[a]	Ethyleneimine[a]
Arsenic[a]	4,4-Methylene(bis)-2 chloronile
Asbestos[a]	Beta-napthylamine[a]
Benzene[a]	Nickel (and salts)
Benzidine[a]	4-Nitrobiphenyl[a]
Bis(chloromethyl) ether[a]	N-Nitrobiphenyl[a]
Chromic acid and chromates[b]	Propiolactone[a]
Coke-oven emissions[a]	Soots, tars, and mineral oils
1,2-Dibromo-3-chloropropane	Vinyl chloride[a]

[a]Permanent standards promulgated after Administrative Procedures Act rulemaking.
[b]From ANSI list.

regulatory scheme that places a burden upon the federal government to prove a process or produce harmful before issuing a regulatory standard. In the 13 years since 1970, OSHA has produced permanent health standards for the regulation of 23 substances. Twenty are carcinogens. Table 2 lists the completed standards.

Table 2 Completed OSHA Permanent Health Standards, as of 1983[a]

Asbestos[b]	14 Carcinogens[b]
Vinyl chloride[b]	Lead
Arsenic[b,c]	Cotton dust
Benzene[b]	1,2-Dibromo-3-chloropropane
Coke-oven emissions[b]	Acrylonitrile[b]

[a]These standards were promulgated following the procedures of Section 6(b) of the OSH Act for the adoption of permanent standards.
[b]Carcinogenic agents.
[c]The arsenic standard was remanded to OSHA by the Court of Appeals for the Ninth Circuit for the purposes of making a significant risk determination consistent with the Supreme Court's benzene decision.

Table 3 Potential Impacts of Selected Chemical Carcinogens in the Workplace[a]

Chemical	Sites of primary cancers	Occupations at risk	1981 NIOSH expected numbers of workers exposed full and part time
Acrylonitrile	Colon, lung	Chemical workers and plastic workers	374,345
Carbon tetrachloride	Liver	Drycleaning, machinists	1,380,232
Ethylene oxide	Leukemia, gastric cancer (suggested)	Hospital workers, laboratory workers, fumigators	144,152
Beryllium	Lung	Beryllium workers, defense and aerospace industry, nuclear industry	855,189
Cadmium	Prostate, respiratory tract, renal	Electrical workers, painters, battery plant and alloy workers	1,376,871
Vinyl chloride	Angiosarcoma-lung, brain, hematopoietic lymphopoietic	Plastics industry	239,375
Arsenic	Skin, lung, liver, lymphatic system	Miners, smelters	255,277

	Cancer sites	Occupations	Amount
		Insecticide makers and sprayers, chemical workers, oil refiners, vintners	432,017 (arsenic oxides)
Asbestos	Lung, pleural, and peritoneal mesothelioma, gastrointestinal tract	Miners, millers, textile, insulation, and shipyard workers	1,280,202
Benzene	Bone marrow (leukemia)	Explosives, benzene, and rubber cement workers, distillers, dye users, printers, shoemakers	1,495,706
Chromium	Nasal cavity and sinuses, lung, larnyx	Producers, processors and users of Cr; acetylene and aniline workers; bleachers; glass, potters, and linoleum workers; battery workers	1,451,631 (oxides)
Nickel	Nasal cavity and sinuses, lung	Nickel smelters, mixers, and roasters, electrolysis workers	1,369,278 (oxides)

[a]Modified from Davis, D. L.: Cancer in the workplace. *Environment. 23*, 30–31 (July/Aug. 1981).

Table 4 Estimates of the Percentage of Total Cancer Associated With Occupation [11]

Preferred estimate	Time period to which estimate applies	Reference
4% U.S. male incidence	1976	12
2% U.S. female incidence	1976	12
6% Male cancers, England	1968–1972	13
2% Female cancers, England	1968–1972	13
15% U.S. male cancers	Not specified	14
5% U.S. female cancers	Not specified	14
23-38% U.S. incidence males[a] and females combined	Near term and future	15
6.8% U.S. male mortality	1977	16
1.2% U.S. female mortality	1977	16

[a]No one preferred estimate given.

Carcinogens adopted under Section 6(a) of the OSH Act are Permanent Standards, too. They are listed in Table 2-1, 29 CFR Part 1900.1000, OSHA General Industry Standards.

It is clear from Table 1 that OSHA has, in its short history as an agency, placed great emphasis on promulgation of standards for chemical carcinogens. Although noone disputes the fact that occupational exposures to certain chemicals and physical agents cause human cancer, there is disagreement about the numbers of workers now affected or who will be in the near future.

Table 3 is a compilation of a variety of estimates of workers exposed to selected chemical carcinogens [10]. Inadequate data, such as lack of information about exposures, make it extremely difficult to estimate occupational exposures even though a number of agents that cause cancer have been identified in the work environment. Table 4 summarizes the estimates of the percentage of total U.S. cancer associated with occupation. A number of studies have addressed the etiology of cancer, including workplace association [11–16].

II. OSHA RULEMAKING PROCEDURES AND METHODS TO ENFORCE A STANDARD FOR A CARCINOGEN

A. Rulemaking to Promulgate a Permanent Health or Safety Standard*

To promulgate a permanent standard, OSHA must adhere to the Federal Administrative Procedures Act of 1956. The specific steps in these proceedings are briefly described below:

1. Advance Notice of Proposed Rulemaking (ANPR)

OSHA publishes in the *Federal Register* its intent to publish a rule. Essentially, this first step in rulemaking is a call for information relating to the subject of the rule. At its discretion, OSHA may hold an Information Hearing to gather relevant data before issuing a proposed rule.

If OSHA judges it to be advantageous, it may appoint an advisory committee to consider the data relating to the proposed rule and charge the committee with making recommendations to the agency. OSHA has not opted for an advisory group since 1974 when considering the Coke Oven Emissions Standard. Appointment of an advisory committee adds about 9 to 12 months to the rulemaking process; legally, such a committee is required to report out in 270 days.

2. Notice of Proposed Rulemaking (NPR)

OSHA publishes the proposed rule in the *Federal Register*. The proposal should represent the agency's best effort with the information at hand. However, it is often alleged that proposed rules are intentionally inept and provocative in order to elicit comments from potential regulatees!

3. Comment Period

Following publication of the proposal, a comment period (usually 60 days) follows for the public to comment on the proposal. If

---

*See Section 6(b), Occupational Safety and Health Act of 1970.

requested by the public, OSHA is obliged to hold a public hearing to air views on the proposal. All OSHA rules for permanent health standards have been associated with hearings.

4. Public Hearings

After *Federal Register* publication of a date, OSHA holds a public hearing presided over by an administrative law judge. Members of the public notify the agency in advance of the hearing that they desire to appear and submit the text or a close text of their remarks. At the hearing, presenters may be questioned by persons recognized by the judge. The hearing record is certified by the judge at the close of the hearing.

5. Posthearing Comment Period

Usually 60 days are allowed for the submission of posthearing comments by the public.

6. Promulgation of the Standard

Although the OSH Act indicates a time period for rule promulgation following the hearing, the courts have ruled that, depending on other responsibilities, the agency has latitude to not adhere to any rigid time frame for rule promulgation. The agency must, however, promulgate on the basis of information in the hearing and comment period. The effective date of a rule is usually established as 60 days from the date of promulgation.

Under Section 6(c)(1) of the Act, OSHA can provide, without regard to the Section 6(b) rule-making procedures described above, for an *emergency temporary standard* (ETS) to take immediate effect upon publication in the *Federal Register*. OSHA must determine that (1) employees are exposed to grave danger from exposure to substances or agents determined to be toxic or physically harmful or form new hazards, and (2) that such emergency standard is necessary to protect employees from such danger. Emergency temporary standards remain in effect no longer than six months after publication. The law requires OSHA to promulgate a permanent standard within this time frame.

An ETS bypasses due process. In general, the courts have not looked kindly upon the ETS procedure, and OSHA has rarely invoked it. As of this writing, OSHA has issued an ETS lowering the asbestos standard [8], however.* It is administratively practically impossible for OSHA to promulgate a permanent standard within the six-month time period following issuance of an ETS, given the size of the task.

B. OSHA Methods to Enforce a Carcinogen Standard

Permanent OSHA standards, as shown above in Table 2 have evolved a common format. The ingredients of these standards will be discussed to indicate the logistical regulatory approach to ensuring that exposures of employees to carcinogens are minimized.

1. Permissible Exposure Limit (PEL)

A concentration of the carcinogenic agent in air which is permissible is defined.† It is usually expressed in terms of agent weight per unit volume of air ($\mu g/m^3$). The PEL is expressed as an average over a time period, i.e., 8 hours, or in some cases there is a supplemental shorter time period. For example, a PEL may also include a short-term exposure limit (STEL) for 15 minutes. It is the obligation of the employer to ensure that all employees are exposed below permissible exposure limits.

2. Action Level

The action level is generally defined as 50% of the PEL. If the average of samples obtained is below the action level, there is a high degree of confidence that the PEL is always met. If the employer maintains exposures below the action level many of the administrative requirements of standards are waived by OSHA.

3. Regulated Zones

Regulated zones are defined as those areas where the material in question is utilized. Regulated zones may be entered only by those requiring access; sign-in/sign-out records are maintained.

---

*Subsequently, the 5th Circuit Court of Appeals remanded the ETS for asbestos.
†No PEL is defined for the "14 carcinogens," Table 2.

4. Engineering Controls

Engineering controls usually include ventilation and specific process requirements.

5. Work Practices

For example, work practices pertain to change of clothing prior to leaving work, showering and washing, methods for cleanup (i.e., vacuum instead of compressed air), and sign-in/sign-out procedures for entry into regulated zones. Some work practices are very specific with regard to cleanup and disposal of the materials.

6. Medical Surveillance

Periodic medical examinations are required. For example, there are requirements for x-rays in the coke-oven emissions and asbestos standards. Pulmonary function tests (asbestos) and sputum cytology (coke oven emissions) are required.

7. Environmental Monitoring

Environmental surveillance or monitoring is required at intervals specified. New employees have a right to an environmental assessment of their workplace within 30 days of employment and a repeat assessment usually every 6 months or annually, depending on the standard. Results of medical and environmental surveillance must be shared with the individual employee and, if specified, the employee's physician or an agent designated by the employee, which could be a union.

8. Labeling and Signs

Signs of very specific wording must be posted in the work area. These signs may take one of the following forms, depending on the standard: "Cancer–Suspect Agent–Authorized Personnel," or "Danger–Cancer Hazard–Authorized Personnel Only." In addition, it may be required that signs be posted for contamination of clothing, required respiratory protective equipment, and limited access.

9. Protective Equipment

Protective equipment required by OSHA standards includes protective clothing, head protection, gloves, and respirators, among
others. The employer must ensure that a program is designed for
periodic maintenance of the equipment, testing of effectiveness of
the equipment (respirators), and employee education and training
in the usage of this equipment. Medical testing is required to ensure that wearing respirators is possible.

10. Education and Training

Employers must ensure that employees understand the nature of
the hazard and the means to deal with it. The employer can use
a variety of methods including classroom and supervisory in-
struction.

C. The Inspection Process

OSHA has the authority to inspect work places for determining
compliance with standards. If requested by the regulatee, the
agency Compliance Safety and Health Officer (CSHO) may have
to obtain an administrative search warrant. In any event, entry to
the premises to inspect has not generally been a problem for
OSHA. The onsite procedure involves a CSHO who holds an
opening conference with the employer and a representative of the
employees, if the latter have such representation. After explaining
the procedures to be followed, the CSHO walks through and observes the facility. Samples of an environment may be collected to
ensure adherence with the appropriate PEL. Samples of the environment are forwarded to an analytical laboratory where the
amount of regulated material collected is determined. In this way
it is possible to calculate the concentrations of the agent in the
environment, expressed as an airborne concentration, to compare
with the PEL. In those cases where conditions in the facility do
not adhere to the standard, the CSHO recommends to the OSHA
area director that a citation be issued to the employer. With concurrence of the OSHA area director, a citation is mailed to the

employer with an associated fine. The employer is also instructed to abate the hazard within a given time and to show interim evidence of progress toward abatement where major changes in the workplace are required, such as engineering controls. The CSHO follows up all serious citations to determine that abatement progress is being made. All citations for carcinogenic agents are by definition designated as serious.

If the employer disagrees with the nature of the citation or the recommended fines, he or she may file an appeal within 15 working days of citation. The appeal will be heard by an administrative law judge. The judge is an agent of the Occupational Safety and Health Review Commission, an administrative agency reporting to the President of the United States and created under the Occupational Safety and Health Act. If the appeal is unsuccessful, the employer has the option of appealing to the district courts and, if necessary, to the Supreme Court. Several OSHA appeals have been adjudicated by the Supreme Court.

It is possible for an employer to obtain a variance from any OSHA standard. The basis for issuance of variances are unavailability or delay in receipt of control equipment. Also, the employer may have utilized a method other than that specified in the standard to achieve control. In this case, it is the responsibility of the employer to prove that the methodology is as effective as that specified by OSHA.

Under the OSH Act, OSHA cannot consult with employers. However, states can offer consultation without citations or penalties. Nearly all states (note: Louisiana does not) now have consultation programs which are funded, for the most part, through funds allocated to OSHA by the Congress.

III. REVIEW OF ACCOMPLISHMENTS OF OSHA TO REDUCE CANCER RISKS

It is not possible to judge the long-term efficacy of OSHA efforts using any measures of health impact because of the long latent period of carcinogenic action. OSHA, as an agency, has been in existence since 1971. The latency period for manifestations of carcinogenicity is, in general, 20 years or more. Therefore, a discussion of the accomplishments of OSHA must be based on surrogate measures of effectiveness. These will be discussed in terms of compliance efforts and reduction of exposure levels of employees exposed to carcinogens on the job.

A. Compliance Efforts

Table 5 displays selective measures of federal OSHA compliance activity for the first half of Federal Year 1983. The data are presented to give some idea of the workers contacted in compliance inspections. Approximately the same number of inspections were conducted by state OSHA programs during the same time period. It can be seen that a total of 26,765 establishments were inspected by federal OSHA during the half-year period, and 4953 health inspections were conducted. Half of the inspection activity was in the construction industry where workers are exposed primarily to noncarcinogens. A total of 1,016,137 employees were covered by

Table 5 Selected Measures of Federal OSHA Compliance Activity for the First Half of FY 1983, as Reported by OSHA

Total inspection	32,093
Records inspections	5,328
Establishment inspections	25,765
New initial inspections	11,605
Repeat initial inspections	14,439
Follow-up	721
Inspections by type	
Safety	21,812
Health	4,953
Inspections by industry	
Construction	15,021
Maritime	372
Manufacturing	9,680
Other	1,692
Employee coverage by inspections	1,016,137

the inspections. If it is assumed that a direct ratio exists between inspections and number of workers, then approximately one-sixth of this total number of workers (or about 175,000) were reached by health inspections. These numbers should be contrasted with the approximately 5 million establishments assigned to OSHA under the Act and the approximately 75 million workers entitled to OSHA protection.

In summary, based on Table 5 data, in an average year OSHA will conduct approximately 64,000 inspections. Of these, about half will be construction and 350,000 workers will receive the benefit of health inspections. These figures, though of recent vintage, reflect a problem OSHA has faced for years; namely, that only a small proportion of workplaces can be inspected in any given year. One can only conclude that the OSHA inspection process cannot have a direct, major impact on reduction of exposure to carcinogens or, for that matter, to any potentially toxic agent in U.S. workplaces.

The establishment of standards does create the requirement for employer compliance with standard ingredients, particularly permissible exposure limits. Most employers do not wish to be in technical violation of the law. Therefore, it is reasonable to assume that at least in the areas that OSHA has promulgated standards, major reductions in exposures have occurred. Although OSHA has only promulgated standards for a few carcinogens, we can examine the impact in selected areas. Table 6 indicates the reduction of exposures to asbestos, as judged by U.S. asbestos standards from 1938 to the present. Once again, if it is assumed that a linear relationship exists between the dose and response to carcinogens, and that exposures to asbestos have, indeed, been reduced from 12 fibers per cc in 1970 to 2 fibers per cc or less in 1983, then OSHA has reduced the future harvest of occupational cancer due to asbestos by five-sixths, or approximately 84%.

In the case of vinyl chloride, 70 U.S. plants employed 940 workers. Forty plants with about 5600 workers produced polyvinyl chloride in 1973 [17]. At that time, exposures apparently varied from 50 to 500 ppm. After promulgation of an OSHA permanent standard for a PEL of 1 ppm in 1974, all of the above

Table 6 U.S. Asbestos Standards

				Million particles/ cm^3	Fibers/ cc	STEL, fibers/ cc
1938	Ref. [19]	Recommended	TLV	5	30[a]	
1946	ACGIH	Adopted		5	30[a]	
1970		Adopted		2	12[a]	
1971		Proposed		–	5	
1971	OSHA	Emergency	TWA	–	2	10
1975		Proposed		–	0.5	5
1976		Adopted		–	2	10
1976	NIOSH	Recommended		–	0.1	0.5
1983	OSHA	ETS			0.5	
1984	OSHA	Proposed		–	0.4 or 0.2	

[a] Approximate fiber equivalent.

employers can be considered to have experienced an exposure reduction of *at least* 98%.

Similar approaches to other carcinogens regulated by OSHA will show the same extraordinary impacts of the standard on the health of workers exposed, when exposure concentration is used as a surrogate measure of subsequent health impact. Using this methodology, it is difficult to predict the future incidence of cancer in exposed populations because of the weaknesses in previous exposure monitoring. It is necessary to assume some average exposure value in the past and, on the basis of dose-response curves, to predict future incidence of cancer. Notwithstanding these limitations, we conclude that in the areas in which permanent health standards have been promulgated, OSHA has had a major impact.

Early in this chapter, the total number of proven or suspect human carcinogens in the workplace was noted. Obviously, the substance-by-substance approach to regulation by OSHA, while effective, has left the majority of such chemicals unregulated. Awareness of the need for more rapid regulation of carcinogens led to development of the OSHA Generic Standard for Carcinogens [7].

B. Generic Carcinogen Standard

Between 1977 and 1980 OSHA made a major effort to promulgate a generic standard for carcinogens. The intent of the effort was to avoid utilizing cumbersome administrative procedures in promulgating permanent standards on a substance-by-substance basis. The generic standard would set up a framework for the regulatory requirements applicable to a given agent once conclusions are reached with regard to its carcinogenicity. The generic standard also offered a schema for reaching conclusions as to carcinogenicity. The standard was promulgated in the last hours of the Carter administration and was remanded by the Reagan administration. It is not displayed as in effect in OSHA General Industry Standards [18]. When one contrasts the number of carcinogenic substances in use and the efforts to promulgate standards for a few now on the OSHA books, the need for a generic cancer standard becomes obvious. If our conclusion that where standards have been promulgated OSHA has been effective in substantially reducing exposures is valid, then what OSHA needs is a more efficient vehicle for promulgating standards. The generic standard would achieve this purpose and should be given a trial. In the absence of additional carcinogenic substances covered by regulation, OSHA's effectiveness will continue to be limited in the context of the total potential cancer problem in U.S. industry.

IV. SUMMARY

Approaches to governmental regulation of carcinogens in the workplace and in the environment have received great emphasis in the United States since the late 1950s. With the exception of the Delaney clause in the Pure Food, Drug and Cosmetic Act, laws and regulations generally attempt to reduce exposures to carcinogens to the lowest feasible or practicable value. Many other nations ban carcinogens; the United States normally does not.

OSHA is the federal agency responsible for the regulation of carcinogens in the workplace. The Administrative Procedures Act of 1956 must be adhered to by this agency in promulgating standards. This is a time consuming and cumbersome procedure. During the period since its formation (1970–1983), the agency has promulgated 23 permanent health standards; 20 of these are for carcinogens. Where a standard has been promulgated, it is concluded that workplace exposures have been dramatically reduced. The desire of employers to be in compliance with the law, coupled with the OSHA inspection process proper, have brought about these reductions in workplace exposures.

Thus, while OSHA efforts are judged to have been successful for a limited number of chemical carcinogens in the workplace, addressed by standards, OSHA cannot be favorably judged if the total number of potential carcinogens in the workplace (about 350) is considered. The recognition of the slow pace of standards development on a substance-by-substance basis led to preparation of the agency generic standard for carcinogens. The latter would establish a framework for control options for any chemical once its classification as a carcinogen was established. This standard would greatly accelerate the promulgation of standards for carcinogens by the agency and has the potential for upgrading OSHA effectiveness in this area. Unfortunately, the standard, after promulgation during the final days of the Carter administration in 1981, has been remanded by the current administration. As of this writing (June 1984), OSHA has not promulgated a permanent standard for a carcinogen since January 1981.

REFERENCES

1. M. Corn, Regulations, standards and occupational hygiene in the U.S. in the 1980's, *Ann. Occ. Hyg. 27 #1*:91–105 (1983).
2. *Toxic Substances Control Act, Registry of Chemicals in Commercial Production*, Office of Toxic Substances, Environmental Protection Agency, Washington, D.C.
3. R. Brickman, S. Jassanoff and T. Illgen, *Chemical Regulation and Cancer: Cross National Study of Policy in Politics*, Final Report, Grant PRA 79-14351, National Science Foundation, Washington, D.C. (November 1982).
4. W. W. Lowrance, *Of Acceptable Risk*, W. Kauffman & Co., Los Altos, CA (1976).

5. Committee on Risk Assessment, *Risk Assessment in the Federal Government: Managing the Process*, National Academy of Sciences, Washington, D.C. (March, 1983).
6. IARC Working Group, *An Evaluation of Chemicals and Industrial Processes Associated with Cancer in Humans Based on Human and Animal Data*. IARC monographs volumes *1-20, Cancer Res. 40*:1-12 (1980).
7. *Identification, Classification and Regulation of Occupational Carcinogens*, Proposal by U.S. Occupational Safety and Health Administration, *Fed. Reg., 42*:54148 (October 4, 1977).
8. Occupational Safety and Health Administration (OSHA), Occupational exposure to asbestos; emergency temporary standard, *Fed. Reg., 48*: 51086-51140 (Nov. 4, 1983).
9. R. Brickman, S. Jassanoff and T. Illgen, *Chemical Regulation and Cancer: A Cross-National Study of Policy and Politics*, p. 144, Program on Sciences, Technology and Society, Cornell University, Ithaca, NY, NSA/PRA 79-143551 (1982).
10. D. L. Davis, Cancer in the workplace, *Environment 23*:30-31 (July/ August, 1981).
11. Office of Technology Assessment, *Assessment of Technologies for Determining Cancer Risks from the Environment*, p. 108, Congress of the United States, Washington, D.C. (1981).
12. E. L. Wynder and G. B. Gori, Guest Editorial: Contribution of the environment to cancer incidence: An epidemiologic exercise, *J. Natl. Cancer Inst., 58*:825-832 (1977).
13. J. Higginson and C. S. Muir, Guest editorial: Environmental carcinogenesis: misconceptions and limitations to cancer control, *J. Natl. Cancer Inst., 63*:1291-1298 (1979).
14. P. Cole, Cancer and occupation: Status and needs of epidemiological research, *Cancer, 39*:1788-1791 (1977).
15. Department of Health Education and Welfare, *Estimates of the Fraction of Cancer in the United States Related to Occupational Factors*, National Cancer Institute, National Institute of Environmental Health Sciences, National Institute of Occupational Safety and Health, Bethesda, MD (1978).
16. R. Doll and R. Peto, The causes of cancer: quantitative estimates of avoidable risks of cancer in the United States today, *J. Natl. Cancer Inst., 66*:1191-1308 (1981).
17. Environmental Protection Agency (EPA), *Scientific and Technical Assessment Report on Vinyl Polyvinyl Chloride*, p. 3, U.S. EPA Office

of Research and Development, Washington, D.C. (600/6-75-004) (December, 1975).

18. Occupational Safety and Health Administration (OSHA), *Safety and Health Standards for General Industry* (29CFR1910), U.S. Dept. of Labor, OSHA 2206, Revised June, 1981, U.S. Supt. Documents, Washington, D.C.

19. W. C. Dreessen et al., A study of asbestos in the asbestos textile industry. U.S. Treasury Department, Public Health Service, *Public Health Bulletin* No. 241, August, 1938.

10

CANCER RISK REDUCTION IN WESTERN EUROPEAN INDUSTRY

Duurt Frederik Rijkels
Shell Internationale Petroleum Maatschappij B.V.
The Hague, The Netherlands

I. INTRODUCTORY REMARKS ON THE PROVISION OF OCCUPATIONAL HEALTH CARE IN WESTERN EUROPE

The problem of control of carcinogenic substances in the workplace is very much in the limelight in most Western European industries. A survey of information on existing legal regulations as well as existing recommendations, agreements, or codes of practice reveals a considerable heterogeneity among the various countries. The structures of legislation and the specific regulations on occupational carcinogens are quite different.

These considerable variances in different European countries are due to historical development, differentiation in the structure of state health care, and differences in political situations which can affect employment conditions.

Occupational health care in most European countries began as a consequence of government-established labor inspectorates where medical advisers were employed to advise on medical problems. Later, larger industries in Europe initiated their own occupational health care systems, often on a voluntary basis, starting generally in the second and third decades of the twentieth century. After World War II, discussions started in European countries on state-controlled occupational health care.

These processes have resulted in legislation and regulation dealing with the working environment and with occupational health in practically every Western European country. This trend began in 1946 in France with the *Code du Travail*, a law encompassing, among other things, the medical surveillance of exposed workers and annual medical or periodic examinations.

Although legislation requires the provision of occupational health care, generally speaking this is primarily a responsibility of the employer in Western European countries, in close collaboration and cooperation with employees. While the government or state authority has a regulatory and controlling function, occupational health care is generally state-controlled but not state-run.

The Permanent Committee of Doctors in the European Economic Community (EEC), an official organization within the EEC, has issued a Charter of Occupational Health on the tasks of industrial medicine in Europe and on the functions of an industrial doctor. This will certainly contribute to greater uniformity in occupational health care, the more so when the EEC directives on the regulation of occupational health care are put into effect.

Professional training for occupational physicians varies from part-time training courses up to three-year, full-time occupational health training.

Quantitatively, from the total working population in the EEC countries of about 115 million people, coverage by occupational health services varies from 40% to 60–70%. Small industry and agriculture are still underserved. Moreover, there is no common epidemiological methodology for evaluating the effect on health of industrial hazards and for the establishment of hygiene standards. In contrast, occupational health care in the United States has developed principally from industrial hygiene practices, importantly influenced by the litigative system; the result has been, in the European view, a rather technical, sometimes defensively colored occupational health care system.

In most European countries there is a considerable State sharing in worker's compensation for industrial injuries or occupational diseases. Compensation is allocated either within the social security system as sickness benefits, or as part of a registered system of industrial injuries or occupational diseases. Consequently, individual claims against employing companies do not occur very frequently in comparison with the United States, and where such claims have been lodged, they often have been settled out of court. This attitude has resulted in a less defensive climate in legal regulations in Western Europe. It has caused the impetus to reach uniform standards or exposure limits, with the possibility of stringency of compliance with (governmental) standards and/or prosecution in different countries, to not be great.

Due to the historical development of occupational health care in the European countries, the present situation has resulted more from the concepts of prevention embodied in social medicine, which are aimed at the social risk of the working population, than from concepts aimed at individual risks combined with compensatory regulations for the individual worker.

The fact that the provision of occupational health care is primarily a responsibility of the employer has led to important accomplishments by industry separate from the requirements of legislation. This has resulted in the establishment by companies of their own toxicological laboratories and of extensive sponsoring of occupational health and toxicological research by industry in independent institutes or laboratories. Position papers on the control and safe handling of chemical carcinogens have been issued either by single large industries or by federations of chemical industries [1-5].

The results of research and the above-mentioned documents are finding use as a basis for discussions with regulatory authorities and with supranational and national organizations and associations.

II. THE ROLE AND THE PROGRAMS OF ACTION OF THE EUROPEAN COMMUNITIES IN THE CONTROL OF OCCUPATIONAL CANCER RISKS

The European communities were established in 1951 and in 1958 as, basically, economic institutions; a number of provisions in the treaties leading to the establishment of these Communities have enabled the European Commission (the European administrative body) to develop actions on health at the community level.

The Council of European Ministers can adopt directives that are legally binding for member States. At the present moment the member States are: The Netherlands, Belgium, Luxemburg,

France, West Germany, Italy, the United Kingdom, Ireland, Denmark, and Greece. The ability to bind members distinguishes the communities from other international organizations which mostly act by means of agreement or conventions that require ratification by member states.

The first European community was the European Coal and Steel Community, established in 1951. Formation of this community permitted the Commission to carry out research and information exchange on occupational health and safety in the coal mining, iron ore mining, and steel making industries.

The community for European cooperation in the field of nuclear energy is called Euratom. This community, in establishing regulations on worker protection, has stated [6] that "the Community shall establish uniform safety standards to protect the health of workers and of the general public and ensure that they are applied." Such safety standards have resulted in a common policy of protection and standardization that has been regularly supplemented and revised, starting in 1959.

The European Commission can work out its policies by the adoption of resolutions and programs of action, and of directives, which are issued by the Council of Ministers of the member States. These administrative practices cover, among other things, restriction of the amounts of controllable exposures, operational protection of exposed workers, and principles for the protection of the population. Thus, a coordinated complex of policies, regulations, and administrative procedures has been established on standard setting; research programs have been initiated as well to validate and support the standards.

The Council of Ministers created the Advisory Committee on Safety, Hygiene and Health Protection at Work in 1974 to assist the European Commission with the preparation of its first Action Program. The composition of this Committee is tripartite (two members from the government, two from employers, and two from workers) representing each member State. In 1978 the Council of Ministers adopted the First Program of Action on Safety and Health at Work [7]. It aimed at improving the protection of all workers within the community.

Among the objectives of the program are: to protect against dangerous substances, to establish a statistical methodology for assessing accidents and the etiology of disease, to improve working situations to increase safety with due regard to health requirements in the organization of the work, to improve knowledge in order to identify and assess risks and to improve prevention and control methods thereby, and to improve human attitudes in order to promote and develop safety and health consciousness. Under this program of action several specific directives have been adopted or proposed: the directive on the protection of the health of workers exposed to vinyl chloride monomer which comprises technical preventive measures, establishment of (technical long-term) limit values for atmospheric concentration of vinyl chloride monomer in the working area of three parts per million, provisions for measuring and monitoring atmospheric concentrations, personal protection measures, guidelines for medical surveillance of workers, and the like; the directive on the protection of workers from harmful exposures to metallic lead and its ionic compounds at work, which includes a time weighted average (TWA) concentration of lead of 150 $\mu g/m^3$ in air, biological parameters for blood, hemoglobin and creatinine, and other values relevant to protective measures; and the directive on the protection of workers from risks related to exposures to agents at work, such as asbestos. Further, a framework directive on the protection of workers from harmful exposures to chemical, physical, and biological agents at work was proposed [8]. The Council agreed that 14 actions could be undertaken up to the end of 1982. Two of these make specific reference to occupational carcinogens. They embody the following actions: to develop a preventive and protective action for substances recognized as being carcinogenic by fixing exposure limits, sampling requirements and measuring methods, by establishing satisfactory conditions of hygiene in the workplace, and by specifying prohibitions where necessary; and to establish information notices on the risks relating to, and handbooks on, the handling of a certain number of dangerous substances such as carcinogenic substances.

In an overall approach to worker protection the most important legal instrument is Directive 80/1107/EEC, adopted by the Council in November 1980, on the protection of workers from the risks related to exposure to chemical, physical, and biological agents at work [8]. The measures established in this directive cover all agents including occupational carcinogens, and thus its application will affect the majority of workers in the community. It will result in member States following a similar legislative path in the future, including short-term and longer-term measures. The short-term measures require that workers and/or their representatives at the place of work receive appropriate information about asbestos, arsenic, cadmium, lead, and mercury; and that there is appropriate health supervision of workers during the period of exposure to asbestos and lead.

The longer-term measures are to be taken by member states to ensure that worker exposure is avoided or kept as low as is reasonably practicable. These measures are to be taken when member states adopt provisions to protect workers against an agent; however, the extent to which each measure applies has to be determined by the member State in question. Fourteen measures can be taken for all agents, plus 5 additional measures for 11 specifically named agents, 7 of which are carcinogens (among them asbestos, benzene, cadmium and compounds, and nickel and compounds). The Council will lay down for these agents, in individual directives, limit values and other specific requirements as applicable.

A second program of action [9] was issued at the end of 1982. In this program the protection of workers against dangerous agents is the first action, indicating the need to develop preventive and protective actions for agents recognized as being carcinogenic. The principles for dealing with carcinogens and other dangerous agents and processes which may produce serious health effects need to be defined and applied, such as fixing exposure limits, defining measuring methods, and determining satisfactory conditions of hygiene at work, and, when necessary, to prohibit use. It is also stated in the second program that an inventory of cancer registers existing at local, regional, and national levels will be compiled with a view to assessing the comparability of the data contained in these registers and to assess the need for better coordination at the community level. The Second EEC Action Program on Health and Safety at Work identifies 20 tasks to be undertaken by the end of 1988.

Further Community rules on carcinogenic substances can be found in the EEC Directive on Dangerous Substances [10]. This directive gives priorities for the classification and labelling of substances according to their hazards. The classification of chemicals as carcinogenic is considered an expert matter, as is the case for mutagenic and teratogenic substances.

III. NATIONAL POLICIES IN SCANDINAVIAN COUNTRIES ON THE PREVENTION OF OCCUPATIONAL CANCER

An important principle in Scandinavian countries is considerable involvement by the workers in the political processes involving final decisions on exposures to carcinogenic substances. Legislation recognizes that it is impossible to achieve complete protection from all carcinogenic hazards at work by removing all carcinogenic substances from the working environment, and that a certain degree of risk has to be accepted in cancer prevention and control. Close collaboration exists between the Nordic countries, although legislative processes take place independently in each country.

The Nordic Council is a supranational organization, founded in 1952 by Denmark, Sweden, Norway, Finland, and Iceland. This Council does not have a legislative status like the EEC, nor can it adopt directives or issue conventions that would need ratification by the individual states. Rather, it has a coordinating role, and as an advisory body, its committees can issue criteria documents, for example, in the field of occupational health.

Carcinogenic risk assessment follows the steps of risk identification and quantitative risk estimation, after which standards are set by the competent authority in collaboration with workers and management. Standards for carcinogenic substances may include:

prohibition; acceptance of use, subject to specific regulations (Code of Practice); or acceptance of general use under the same conditions as for other chemicals with limitation on the level of exposure.

Regulatory agencies, legislation, and the health care systems of the countries control the actual use of the substances and the surveillance of the workers. Registries of exposed workers linked to general cancer registries exist in Scandinavian countries. For example, in Finland a government decree obliges employers annually to inform the authorities about the use of carcinogens and the workers exposed. The general objectives of registration are to increase the rates of identification and evaluation of carcinogens, and to stimulate preventive measures in the workplace. The linkage of the computerized data with the Finnish Cancer Registry in the future will provide information on cancer incidence according to carcinogen, occupation, industry, and region. The definition of exposure in practical situations forms a difficulty in this recently established system. A list of 50 carcinogens is currently in use [11], and will soon be expanded to 162 carcinogens.

IV. OTHER IMPORTANT INTERNATIONAL ORGANIZATIONS IN EUROPE

A. Conseil Européen des Fédérations de l'Industrie Chimique (CEFIC)

The European Council of Chemical Manufacturers Federations (CEFIC) permits its members to develop coordinated approaches to topics of common interest, and to utilize expertise and experience to achieve a common view. This enables CEFIC to speak with authorities on behalf of the Western European Chemical Industry. There is coordination of effort on matters of occupational health, safety, and the protection of the environment. CEFIC has established four main committees and ancillary task forces, among which the Health Protection Committee deals with the provision of advice and guidance on health protection matters and the risk assessment of chemical substances.

CEFIC issued a position paper on the control of occupational carcinogens [1], supporting the EEC Framework Directive and calling for establishing common procedures for the identification and classification of carcinogenic substances. This will eventually result in an estimate of the carcinogenic potency of substances in pure form as well as in dilutions and lead to scientifically advised exposure limits for the workplace and possibly to other relevant factual recommendations.

B. European Chemical Industry Ecology and Toxicology Centre (ECETOC)

The European Chemical Industry Ecology and Toxicology Centre (ECETOC) is an organization of chemical companies in Western Europe concerned with the scientific aspects of toxicity and ecology. It comprises 40 companies who have pooled their expertise, experts, and experience to assess the potential hazards of their products, and thus to exchange information on test methods and methodology to avoid costly duplication.

The Centre procures information relevant to the protection of the health of persons who come into contact with chemicals. It operates in scientific contact with governments, health authorities, and all other public institutions concerned with ecological and toxicological problems relating to chemicals. Members are drawn from all Western European companies, including some major U.S. companies with operations in Europe. ECETOC has published important monographs on occupational carcinogens, both on the identification and control and on the risk assessment of occupational chemical carcinogens [12, 13]. In these monographs, concise definitions of carcinogenic potential, risk, and potency are given and carcinogens are defined in four categories: (1) proven human chemical carcinogens, (2) putative human chemical carcinogens, (3) questionable human chemical carcinogens, and (4) human chemical noncarcinogens.

Carcinogenic risk assessments are made using a three-step procedure to avoid the danger of equating carcinogenic potential with carcinogenic risk. These three steps are:

1. Hazard Identification

This is necessary to identify chemicals by classifying them, using all available evidence, according to the definitions given above.

2. Quantitative Risk Estimation

Even with proven human chemical carcinogens, quantitative risk estimation is only relatively straightforward when the duration and intensity of exposure are known. With putative and questionable human chemical carcinogens, the quantitative estimation of the carcinogenic potential is difficult because no adequate human data are available and qualitative information is incomplete. The risk quantification takes into consideration an assessment of exposure after having established the anticipated carcinogenic potential of the substance in man, the hazard assessment.

3. Risk Evaluation and Limitation

When the risk identification and quantification have been carried out, the acceptability of risk to society is the next crucial point. This involves ranking of the anticipated cancer risk on the scale of other recognized risks and balancing it against society's willingness to accept the risk. Social benefit, economic cost of control of exposure and available technology need to be taken into account. The end result of this stage is the development of recommendations governing exposure conditions, the handling of the carcinogen, and any other measures necessary to ensure that the risk is controlled to a suitably low level by means which are technologically feasible and take into account the social and economic consequences of the proposals. Risk limitation should be considered by a group in which the parties ultimately concerned with implementing the recommendations made to control the risk are represented, plus experts from the risk estimation group.

This three-stage process is an important philosophy that has had great influence on several governmental regulations and recommendations, for example, in the United Kingdom, The Netherlands, Belgium, and the Scandinavian countries.

C. International Agency for Research on Cancer (IARC)

The IARC was established in 1965 by the World Health Organization's (WHO) World Health Assembly as an independently financed organization within the framework of WHO. The headquarters of the Agency are at Lyon, France, and it has research centers outside of Europe.

The Agency conducts programs of research concentrating particularly on the epidemiology of cancer and the study of potential carcinogens in the human environment. Its field studies are supplemented by biological and chemical research, carried out in the Agency's laboratories in Lyon and through collaborative research agreements in national research institutions in many countries. The Agency also conducts programs for the education and training of personnel for cancer research. Among the publications of the Agency are Monographs on the Evaluation of the Carcinogenic Risk of Chemicals to Humans, Volumes 1–29.

D. British Industrial Biological Research Association (BIBRA)

The British Industrial Biological Research Association (BIBRA) is a research institute and laboratory for the British food and pharmaceutical industry. BIBRA has played a major role in toxicological research on food additives and in providing information to industry. Since 1982 BIBRA has been expanding its activities to include industrial chemicals. It has played a liaison role in cooperation with expert committees of the British government.

E. Other Organizations

Space does not permit the full listing, much less the full description, of all relevant organizations. Some of the other national or supranational industrial organizations that are influential in research activities or making recommendations on carcinogenic substances are: the Association of Plastics Manufacturers in Europe (APME); the major oil companies' international study group for Conservation of Clean Air and Water in Europe (CONCAWE); the

International Isocyanate Institute (III); and the International Institute of Synthetic Rubber Producers (IISRP).

V. NATIONAL REGULATIONS ON OCCUPATIONAL CARCINOGENS

The Western European countries are each very much interested in control of carcinogenic substances in the workplace and they observe the resolutions and the programs of action. EEC member States, moreover, are legally bound to follow directives of the Council of Ministers of the European Communities. Nonetheless, there is still much heterogeneity among the various national regulations on occupational carcinogens: the legislative structures vary as do the substances regulated.

Certain substances can be regulated in states as carcinogens or otherwise; in either case, threshold limit values (TLV) or maximum accepted concentrations (MAC) requirements must be met. Both TLV and MAC values are published in Austria, Denmark, the Federal Republic of Germany, the Netherlands, Sweden, Switzerland, and the United Kingdom. In France the TLV lists of United States and the Soviet Union are published as a reference by the *Institute National de Recherche et Sécurité*. In Italy the TLV list of the United States is published.

Legal provisions for the control of carcinogens vary from country to country and, complementary to legislation, there may be tripartite agreements between government, employees, and employers on control limits. Observance of MAC or TLV values by measurement of exposures is required but is seldom enforced by legal requirements. In some countries the labor inspectorate can enforce certain norms within an industry.

In the United Kingdom the Health and Safety Committee (HSC) was set up by the Secretary of State to advise on health and safety at the same time as the Health and Safety Executive (HSE) approved a Code of Practice, still in draft form, entitled "Control of Carcinogenic Substances" in accordance with Section 16 of the Health and Safety at Work etc. Act of 1974. The Code of Practice gives supplementary practical guidance with respect to regulations

on substances hazardous to health and should be read in conjunction with the already generally approved Code of Practice, "Control of Substances Hazardous to Health." These codes of practice
were drawn up on the basis of joint discussions between representatives of the Confederation of British Industry, the Trade
Union Congress, the local authorities, government departments, independent experts, and the HSE.

Although failure to comply with any provision of this United
Kingdom code is not in itself an offense, that failure may be used
in criminal proceedings. The code applies for persons who are exposed and who are liable to be exposed to the carcinogenic substances named in its paragraphs. It gives guidance on assessments
needed to determine whether or not substances to which this code
relates are present in a workplace; also, control measures are
spelled out and guidelines for selecting personal protective equipment are given. Monitoring programs should be established and
used to determine the extent of exposure to individuals, to detect
any departure from standards, and to help assess the degree of
benefit from any improved control measures. Monitoring should
be carried out frequently or continuously, as appropriate, and
records should be kept.

This use of a Code of Practice does not exist in other European
countries.

In the Federal Republic of Germany (FRG) a practical approach in regulating carcinogens is in use. A basic intent of the approach is to limit the use or dissemination of carcinogens in the
environment.

For the Federal Republic of Germany, of MAK Commission
(maximum permissible concentration) observes the following categories: A1, or human carcinogens; A2, or proven animal carcinogens; and B, or suspect carcinogens for which further research is
needed. Substances categorized as A1 and A2 are given a
Technische Richt Konzentration or Technical Guiding Concentration (TRK) in which the following subcategories are set: highly
dangerous, very dangerous, and dangerous. Guidelines are given in
the handling of these carcinogens. A separate commission of the
Ministry of Labor sets these TRK values, for which no MAK values

are known due to a lack of adequate toxicological occupational evaluation.

In principal, both the A1 and A2 substances are all carcinogens. The TRK is a concentration in air to be used as a guideline for protection and for measurement strategy in the workplace. Observing the TRK reduces the risk, but does not necessarily exclude it. The TRKs are on a yearly average basis. Differentiation of approach for specific controlling of carcinogens is attained by the categorization into subgroups I, II, and III of the categories A1 and A2. This allows further specific regulation of each of these groups and assists in assessing the cancer risk due to workplace exposures. Subgroup III contains substances for which it is assumed that a carcinogenic effect for humans is improbable; substances in subgroup III can be used freely if the TRK is observed and exposure is as low as possible. Where necessary, personal protection gear may be used. For subgroup II it is necessary to obtain a governmental use registration and to submit a specific review file containing the relevant properties of the substance, in addition to the regulations for subgroup III. Furthermore, it is necessary to register the workers exposed, the modes of handling and, in general, the preventive measures. Requirements for subgroup I include those for subgroups III and II; in addition, one has to prove that a substitute cannot be used on technical grounds, that a less dangerous substance cannot be used technically, and that the maximum working time is 6 hours per day, 30 hours per week [14].

VI. CANCER REGISTRATION DATA

In most European countries there are state-run cancer registries. The United Kingdom, Denmark, Finland, Norway, Iceland, and Sweden have national cancer registries, whereas in the Federal Republic of Germany, France, and Italy there are regional cancer registries, but no availability on a national basis. In the Netherlands and Belgium mortality statistics are available, but no specific cancer registration is possible because of privacy legislation under the EEC recommendations. In countries that have national cancer registry organizations, there is usually a division into regions that

handle cancer information, each region providing a central coordinating system with minimum information on personal data,
primary site of cancer, histology (if available), and the date of
diagnosis. Privacy of the individual in these countries is guarded by
central ethics committees that have agreed to a national cancer
registration scheme and that will, where necessary, release data on
cancer registration to the central organization as long as appropriate restraints are observed. Upon request, for certain specific research projects, the data can be made available to industrial
doctors.

Registration data are made available from hospitals and out–patient departments but not from general practitioners. In practice
this means that in most countries a significant amount of data can
be made available.

In all countries the identification of carcinogenic potential takes
place via epidemiological methods, animal studies, and short term
predictive tests for carcinogenic activity. It should be realized,
however, that within the 10 member States of the EEC mortality
data are easy to obtain in only two countries, with considerable
difficulty in two others, and that in the remaining countries there
are legal obstacles to obtaining mortality diagnoses of individuals
because of the above mentioned privacy legislation.

The generally limited information on exposure or occupation
over the whole of the latency period before the appearance of cancer restricts the value, due to lack of precision, of most epidemiological studies. Still they remain an essential method for evaluating
the carcinogenicity of chemicals already in use, preferably combined with the presently available methods of cancer registration.

VII. CONCLUSIONS

The reduction of cancer risk in Western European Industry is
complicated in some respects by the diversity of the separate
governmental approaches as compared, say, to the governing federal approach taken in the United States. Nonetheless, through
forceful international cooperative efforts combined with national
governmental systems and reinforced by industry's voluntary

efforts, significant progress has been made and more will be forth-coming. A strength of the Western European system may well be the frequent abilities of government, labor, scientific experts, and management to agree on new standards in nonconfrontational ways. Thus, new standards can be developed and put into place more readily, affording early improved protection to those poten-tially exposed to carcinogenic hazards.

REFERENCES

1. *CEFIC Position Paper on the Control of Occupational Carcinogens*, pp. 1-6, European Council of Chemical Manufacturers Federation (CEFIC), Brussels, Belgium (1982).
2. *Principles for the Safe Handling of Mutagens, Carcinogens and Terato-gens*, Report Series MED/TOX 80.001, Shell International Research Maatschappij B.V., The Hague, Netherlands (1980).
3. J. L. Greig, *Guidelines on the Prevention of Occupational Ill-Health from Chemical Carcinogens in the Workplace*, pp. 1-7, Ciba-Geigy (UK) Lim-ited, London (1981).
4. *The Regulation of Occupational Carcinogens—A CBI Policy Statement*, pp. 1-5, Confederation of British Industry, Centre Point, London (1983).
5. *The Control of Occupational Carcinogens*, pp. 1-12, The Reports of an Ad Hoc Working Group, Chemical Industries Association, London (1981).
6. Council Directive of 15 July 1980, *Official Journal of the European Com-munities*, No. *L246* (Sept. 17, 1980); [Original Directive published in *Official Journal of the European Communities*, No. 11, (Feb. 2, 1959)].
7. Council Resolution of 29 June 1978 on an Active Programme of the European Communities on Safety and Health at Work, *Official Journal of the European Communities*, No. *C165* (July 11, 1978).
8. Council Directive of 27 November 1980 on the Protection of Workers from the Risks Related to Exposure to Chemical, Physical, and Biological Agents at Work, *Official Journal of the European Communities*, No. *L327* (December 3, 1980).
9. Proposal for a Council Resolution on the Second Programme of Action of the European Communities on Safety and Health at Work, *Official Journal of the European Communities*, No. *C308* (November 25, 1982).

10. EC Directive on the Approximation of the Laws, Regulations, and Administrative Provisions Relating to the Classification, Packaging and Labelling of Dangerous Substances, *Official Journal of the European Communities*, p. 1, No. *196* (August 16, 1967) [amended by Council Directive of September 18, 1979, *Official Journal of the European Communities*, No. *L259* (October 25, 1979)–for the last time adapted on July 29, 1983, *Official Journal of the European Communities*, No. *L257* (September 16, 1983)].

11. *Resolution of the Ministry of Social Affairs and Health on Substances to be Considered Cancer Risks and their Markings and Poison Classifications (1063/83)*, Helsinki, Finland (December 21, 1983).

12. *A Contribution to the Strategy for the Identification and Control of Occupational Carcinogens*, Monograph No. 2, European Chemical Industry Ecology and Toxicology Centre (ECETOC), Brussels (September, 1980).

13. *Risk Assessment of Occupational Chemical Carcinogens*, Monograph No. 3, European Chemical Industry Ecology and Toxicology Centre (ECETOC), Brussels (January, 1982).

14. *Maximale Arbeitsplatzkonzentrationen und Biologische Arbeitsstoff-Toleranzwerte 1983*, Deutsche Forschungsgemeinschaft (DFG), Bonn (1983)–[English translation available].

11

SCIENCE, POLICY, AND THE LAW: A DEVELOPING PARTNERSHIP IN REDUCING THE RISK OF CANCER

Robert C. Barnard
Cleary, Gottlieb, Steen and Hamilton, and
American Industrial Health Council
Washington, D.C.

I. INTRODUCTION

It is common to speak of law and science as opposites. Law, it is said, is adversarial and legal disputes are resolved through one-sided presentations of the best facts by an advocate for each side. The scientific approach, on the other hand, seeks consensus based on an evaluation of all the facts with rational impartiality.

These generalizations gloss over the respects in which law and science are basically comparable. Both law and science deal with probabilities. The law uses terms such as "preponderance of the evidence" or "proof beyond a reasonable doubt," terms which are counterparts to the probabilistic terminology of the scientist. And both law and science use the weight of the evidence or the probability criteria to reach decisions and determine causality in specific cases.

In the case of cancer, the time between initiation and the visible onset of disease—the latency period—may be long, up to years or decades. This fact makes the determination of causation difficult.

The development of an interaction or "partnership" between law and science stems from the need of an adequate science base to determine cause in the legal sense. The most significant development of this partnership has occurred in the regulation by government of factors affecting health and the environment. This development is evolutionary, and though it has roots that go back a long way in time, particularly in the regulation of drugs and food, the partnership has developed largely during the last two decades and has focused mainly on carcinogenesis. This chapter will review the progress made to date in several regulatory areas and the possibilities for improvement in adapting science and law to measure, manage, and control the risks of cancer from industrially produced substances.

II. THE BACKGROUND OF AN EVOLVING
   PARTNERSHIP

There are three factors that form the background for the evolving partnership. First, there is the mounting evidence of some carcinogenic activity and hence a potential carcinogenic risk from an

increasingly large list of substances. Second, it is helpful to understand the complementary role of the scientist and the regulator
under the law and the distinction between the scientific evaluation
of risk and the societal decision on how to manage the risk. In the
past, it was common to ask the toxicologist to identify a "safe"
level for a particular substance. This was a natural request made
before it became clear that "safe" involved a societal judgment of
acceptability—a judgment based in part on science but nonetheless
societal rather than scientific. Third, the law has a long tradition
against dealing with trivialities. In the *Benzene* case the Supreme
Court interpreted the Occupational Safety and Health Act to
apply only to "significant" occupational risks of cancer and to
authorize an occupational standard only when the standard would
"significantly" reduce the risk of cancer [1]. Similarly, the federal
Court of Appeals recently held that the prohibition in the Delaney
Clause (forbidding intentional food additives that are shown by
appropriate tests to cause cancer in man or animals) did not apply
to those "de minimis" situations which clearly present no health
or safety concerns [2]. Science figures in the application of the
legal aversion toward making decisions on trivialities.

A.   The Growing Evidence of Potential Cancer Risk

The science of carcinogenesis is a young and rapidly developing
science. In a recently published interview [3] Dr. David Rall, Director of the National Toxicology Program, commented: "We are
dealing with a science that is only two decades old."

Indeed, it was as late as 1954 when the first department combining toxicology, medicine, and basic research in the life sciences
leading to the Ph.D./M.D. degree was established [4] at New York
University, and industry and other universities have since established similar facilities. In government, the National Animal Bioassay Program (the predecessor to the National Toxicology
Program) to test potential carcinogens had its origins in programs
initiated by the National Cancer Institute in the 1960s [5]. The
bioassay program in its present form was launched in a significant
way only in the early 1970s, at the time the "war on cancer" was
declared.

The tremendous increase in research in government, academic, and industrial laboratories has resulted in a rapidly growing mass of evidence relating to potential risks of cancer. By 1976, a National Institute of Occupational Safety and Health (NIOSH) report on potential carcinogens listed literature references for some 1500 substances for which there were experimental results that raised questions of potential carcinogenic risk [6]. This list of substances for which there is *some* evidence of carcinogenic activity in *some* test system at *some* dose is now available in computer form and continues to grow each year by the addition of 300 to 400 additional substances.

The experimental identification of an ever increasing number of substances with some carcinogenic activity generates a mounting need for scientific evaluation of the data relevant to potential chronic health hazards. The number of substances in our air, water, and food for which there are some signals of carcinogenic activity multiplies daily. There is no "easy out" to this problem, for many of these substances for which there is evidence of carcinogenic potential from experimental data at high doses are essential to human life, e.g., hormones and certain vitamins and trace minerals. The magnitude of the problem was illustrated dramatically by the FDA in 1979. FDA responded to a proposal to provide a label warning of all detectable carcinogenic substances in food, thus:

> Indeed, a requirement for warnings on all foods that may contain an inherent carcinogenic ingredient or a carcinogenic contaminant (*in contrast to a deliberately added carcinogenic substance*) would apply to many, perhaps most, foods in a supermarket. (44 *Fed. Reg.* 59509, 59513, October 16, 1979) (emphasis added).

The increase in research already noted and the need for evaluation has resulted in the development of rules by some agencies to provide reasonable assurance of the integrity or the sturdiness and reliability of experimental data. The Food and Drug Administration (FDA) and the Environmental Protection Agency (EPA) have adopted Good Laboratory Practice (GLP) rules and inspection procedures. These rules apply only to tests that are submitted as the basis of a determination by EPA or FDA. Nonetheless, sturdiness of data is a consideration beyond the cases where GLP applies. The National Toxicology Program announced the withdrawal from publication of a report of a bioassay because the discovery of significant discrepancies in the experimental data obtained by a contractor compromised the interpretation of the data [7]. Following this discovery, new audit procedures were instituted to prevent such experimental flaws [8].

Problems of evaluation arise not only because of the mass of experimental data and questions of their validity, but also because the interpretation of the data is ultimately judgmental. A well-known example is nitrites. The original bioassay was reported to be positive; great public uproar and regulatory activity took place because nitrites are important antibacterial additives to meat. Upon full peer review of the data, the study was judged to be negative.

Similarly, a review by a committee of the Society of Toxicology (SOT) of the histopathology in the "megamouse" ED_{01} study involving more than 24,000 female mice highlighted the judgmental aspect of interpreting experimental results. The SOT review of tissue slides for 4000 mice resulted in major disagreement (tumor or no tumor) in 5% to 12% of the slides and some disagreement in some 30% of the slides [9]. In other cases, the Food and Drug Administration (FDA) has approved color additives because on review of the slides FDA differed from the investigator in its interpretation of the data [10] or reevaluated the studies in light of tumor incidence in historical controls [11].

When the law faces the critical question of cause or causation, an evaluation is essential to an understanding of the nature and magnitude of the risk and especially of its relevance to humans. Whether the issue of human risk arises in the legislature considering new laws, or in a regulatory agency trying to reduce and control cancer risks, or in litigation to determine responsibility for injury, the history of the last two decades points to the growing realization that scientific evaluation of the data relevant to chronic health hazards is critical to sensible social decisions. Moreover, insights from new research open new horizons of investigation and impact the scientific evaluation of chronic health hazards. The partnership of law and science to deal with cause and causation must be structured to assure not only the adequacy of the science base but that the latest available science is taken into account as a basis for regulatory decisions.

B. Scientific Risk Assessment and Societal Risk Management

To define the appropriate role of science in the legal context, it is important to distinguish between the function of scientific risk assessment and the regulatory function of risk management. The recent report of the National Academy of Sciences (NAS) [12] provides a useful description of that distinction: *risk assessment* involves the scientific evaluation of data and the characterization of the risk, while *risk management* involves the integration of scientific risk assessment with broad social and political statutory objectives to decide whether and how to regulate.

The NAS Report describes four parts of the scientific risk assessment: (1) *hazard identification*: gathering and evaluating experimental and other data; (2) *dose response assessment*: evaluating the magnitude of the response in relation to the magnitude of exposure; (3) *exposure assessment*: scientific evaluation of data; and (4) *risk characterization*: judgmental integration of all the data to evaluate the probability and magnitude of human risk.

Risk management involves a determination of the social significance of the risk identified by the scientific risk assessment and a determination of the appropriate response. These management decisions are made by government and by industry. In the regulatory context, these decisions are within the regulatory function; this is the area of the lawyer and the regulator.

Risk in the scientific context refers to the evaluation and characterization described above. The term "risk" has also been commonly associated with "risk/benefit," and some erroneously assume that assessing risk implies risk/benefit evaluation. Scientific risk assessment supplies one ingredient of a risk/benefit evaluation, and where such an evaluation is appropriate, science may also be involved in the scientific assessment of benefits. However, the risk/ benefit balancing or the risk/risk balancing (as in the case of a cancer drug which may itself be a carcinogen) is part of the risk management social decision and not of the scientific risk assessment process.

In simple terms, science is a tool which a regulator uses to assist in making the difficult legal and societal judgments required by law. The regulator must decide if the risk characterized in the scientific risk assessment is societally significant and whether the threat of injury is sufficiently important to justify regulation. In some cases, the regulator considers benefits. These are societal, legal judgments. They utilize the underlying scientific assessment, but are not in themselves scientific.

1. Social Policy Distinguished from Science Policy

The NAS report speaks of "policy" in the context of both scientific risk assessment and risk management. The foregoing discussion pointed out the role of the scientific evaluation as a basis for regulatory decisions that implement broad social policy objectives in the law. To serve that purpose, the scientific assessment must be impartial, objective and complete, and must disclose uncertainties in the analysis. The NAS report points out that the scientific analysis will involve analytic choices by the scientist in the assessment process. These choices, the NAS concluded, involve both scientific and "policy" considerations.

To explain what scientific policy considerations are, the NAS Report analyzes the steps in a scientific risk assessment and describes some of the option choices in each step. For example, in evaluating epidemiologic data the scientists must decide what weight should be given studies with different results. Another example is the degree of confirmation of a positive animal study and the relevance of comparative metabolic data in evaluating the results. Choices among the analytic options involve *science policy*, which is different in character from the *social policy* used in making regulatory decisions.

The fact that science policy determinations are made in the course of a scientific evaluation, however, should not be an excuse to inject economic and social policies into the scientific analysis. Neither economic or political judgments nor a scientist's personal value judgments should affect or constrain the scientific evaluation. The scientific evaluation should be unbiased, objective, and free of constraints imposed by management policy dictates.

It is sometimes said that the scientific evaluation of risk should be "conservative" because it deals with human health. But this puts "conservatism" in the wrong place in the regulatory structure. It is the function of the regulator to apply the social criteria of cost, safety, reasonableness, and acceptability. It is in making these decisions that "conservatism" may play a role. If a scientific evaluation is constrained in the name of "conservatism" by social values or management policy, the result will be biased in unobvious ways. Such an evaluation does not provide a sound basis for the difficult social/legal decisions a regulator must make.

EPA Administrator Ruckelshaus, in a recent major policy speech before the National Academy of Sciences, stressed the importance of an adequate science base for regulatory decisions [13]. His speech contrasted regulatory decisions based on social policies with scientific evaluation which must be free of bias and be unconstrained by sociopolitical "policies":

> Scientists assess a risk to find out what the problems are. The process of deciding what to do about the problems is risk management.
>
> •
>
> Despite these often conflicting pressures, risk assessment at EPA must be based on scientific evidence and scientific consensus *only*. Nothing will erode public confidence faster than the suspicion that policy considerations have been allowed to influence the assessment of risk. (Emphasis in the original text.)

A scientific assessment should be neither "conservative" nor "liberal." The assessment must be objective; science "policy" judgments should not be a device to inject social policy constraints.

2. Scientific Extrapolation: Mathematical Models

The scientific evaluation of a carcinogenic potential should involve an examination of the validity and relevance of all the data—toxicological, epidemiological, exposure, comparative metabolism, and pharmacokinetic—to characterize the human risk. Since the evaluation involves probabilities, to be most useful it should provide "most likely" or "most probable" values or estimates [14]. While worst case or upper limit values may also be developed and reported, it is well to remember that worst case risk assessments do not predict actual risk; to the contrary, as the Food and Drug Administration reminded us [15]:

> [U]pper limit estimates of risks using "worst case" assumptions cannot be used to predict with mathematical precision what will actually occur. . . . *"[W]orst case estimates"* . . . *are factored in to reach a conclusion* with reasonable *certainty of what will not occur.* (Emphasis added.)

Much of the discussion of the use of science in decision making regarding potential cancer risks revolves around the use of mathematical models for evaluating carcinogenic responses to various doses (or, dose response) in scientific risk assessment. This is not the place to discuss the extensive literature on this subject (the NAS Report [12] provides an extensive list of references), but it is important to understand the basic uncertainties and inadequacies involved in these procedures when considering science, regulation, and the law.

Dose response assessment and the risk characterization steps in risk assessment normally involve two extrapolation procedures when experimental data are used. First, the response must be extrapolated from high experimental doses to the low levels to which humans are normally exposed; and second, the predicted response at low doses must be extrapolated across species from the experimental data to predict human risk. Both extrapolation procedures may involve the use of models. Dose response mathematical models are formulas subjected to statistical procedures to assist the evaluating scientist, not a separate risk assessment

discipline. Models merely provide statistical evaluation of dose response relationships or formal methods for extrapolating across
species.

Dose response models do not yet deal with the full range of experimental data nor are models yet developed to handle the full
complexity of extrapolation across species. Cross species extrapolation is based on assumptions of comparative sensitivity, and
most low dose extrapolation models are based on very broad assumptions about mechanisms of carcinogenesis. While these assumptions may in some cases appear to have a biological basis in
theory, they are not, in fact, biologically or experimentally validated. The dose response models do not incorporate comparative
pharmacokinetics nor take into account repair and detoxification
processes which occur at the cellular level, either for high-to-low
dose or interspecies extrapolation. Even though a metabolic
change might be required to convert a substance into a carcinogenic form, the dose delivered to the target organ is assumed to be
proportional to the administered dose. Hoel et al. have recently
urged that extrapolation would be more meaningful if the models
were based on delivered dose to the target cell rather than on the
administered dose levels. Models currently used potentially overestimate risk by several orders of magnitude when nonlinear
kinetics are present [16].

Different assumptions can change the results of extrapolations
to very low doses by several orders of magnitude. The models
commonly used by the regulatory agencies differ but normally involve several fundamental assumptions: the exposed person is exposed for a full lifetime at the specified level; competing mortality
risks are disregarded and the model is constructed so that all
events predicted occur at one point in time (age 72); linearity at
low dosage levels, i.e., that the effect is directly proportional to
the dose; and an assumption as to the relative sensitivity of man as
compared to the experimental animals.

During the Occupational Safety and Health Administration
(OSHA) hearing to modify the permissible occupational exposure
limit for ethylene oxide (EtO) from 50 ppm on an 8-hour time
weighted average (TWA) to 1 ppm TWA, Dr. Kenneth Crump, who

designed the computer program for the mathematical model used by EPA, the Consumer Product Safety Commission (CPSC), and OSHA, testified that the exposure assumptions incorporated in the models are unrealistic [17]:

> It should be kept in mind that the exposure scenarios considered probably do not approximate the exposure of any significant population of workers. Risks were estimated from continuous exposure for 45 years, and probably only a tiny fraction of the total work force exposed to EtO would have exposures which approached this in duration. Also, risks from exposures to 1 ppm (say) should not be equated with risks that would accrue under a 1 ppm standard. In order to achieve compliance with a 1 ppm standard, long term TWA exposures would necessarily be less than 1 ppm.

Statistical/mathematical models can *assist* the scientist in evaluation. However, dose response models use only one biological observation—tumor incidence—and deal only with the dose-response function in relation to this incidence. Pharmacokinetic data and other observations such as detoxification and repair and data on mechanisms are relevant to dose response evaluation as well.

Dr. Robert Squire (a distinguished Johns Hopkins cancer scientist) in a recent exchange of letters in *Science* with Dr. Crump emphasized this point [18]:

> As indicated by Crump, a weakness of the model-fitting approach is the lack of information at low dose exposure. However, a greater weakness as indicated above, is that models ignore much of the relevant biological information derived from animal tests. I am not opposed to the use of models. However, they are currently based on too limited data, and *I would prefer their use in conjunction with the weight of biological evidence.* (Emphasis added.)

A workshop organized by the National Center for Toxicological Research and the Society of Toxicology reviewed the statistical implications of the ED_{01} (megamouse) study, already mentioned, for risk assessment [19]. That seminar reviewed not only the massive ED_{01} data base but also a number of other large scale studies. A major consensus conclusion of the workshop was that:

Development of better models for low-dose extrapolation can be aided by the incorporation of more biological information, such as pharmacokinetics, metabolism, and comparative physiology.

A scientific evaluation for carcinogenic risk is complex. It should include not only tumor incidence (and the results of modeling), but also information on, among other things, mechanisms, pharmacokinetics, comparative metabolism, and tumor type and its relevance to humans. As Squire has pointed out, negative and positive data should be assessed [20] and epidemiological data should be evaluated when available. A full scientific evaluation necessarily involves informed examination of the validity, relevance, and sturdiness of all the data and a judgmental evaluation to characterize the risk quantitatively and to state the uncertainties. Failure to include such considerations can result not only in a faulty risk assessment, it can influence court decisions against regulations based on such decisions. A case in point is that of formaldehyde.

3. An Example: The Formaldehyde Case

The limited utility of a risk assessment based on modeling and a consideration of only part of the data provided part of the foundation for the recent decision of the United States Court of Appeals for the Fifth Circuit in the *Formaldehyde* case [21]. The case is noteworthy because it discussed what scientific data and conclusions are essential to a determination of whether there is substantial evidence to support regulatory conclusions. In short, the court dealt with the role science plays in the determination of risk (causation) which becomes the basis for regulatory action.

The *Formaldehyde* case involved a ban by the Consumer Product Safety Commission of urea formaldehyde foam insulation in homes and schools. CPSC found that exposure to formaldehyde gas emitted by the foam created an unreasonable hazard of acute injury and an unreasonable risk of cancer.

In *Formaldehyde*, CPSC had negative epidemiologic data (which both the agency and the court agreed were inconclusive) and three sets of experimental data: two rat studies and one mouse study. CPSC selected Global 79, a computer program of a mathematical model also used by EPA and, in a modified form, by OSHA. The court showed a sophisticated understanding of the model when it stated that:

> Unlike some other models, Global 79 does not predict an actual or most likely risk. Rather it predicts a range of risk within which there is a 95% possibility the actual risk will fall. (at p. 1141.)

CPSC, following another fairly standard regulatory practice, selected the experimental data which gave the highest risk estimate to use with Global 79 (a practice also followed by EPA).

The court criticized the CPSC methodology on two grounds: first, CPSC's reliance on one animal data base and failing to analyze the other data bases available, and second, the use of upper confidence limit values, both with respect to evaluation of acute hazard from formaldehyde exposure and for extrapolation of cancer risk. On the second point, the court commented that such findings provide no basis for review under the substantial evidence standard.

The court also noted other issues regarding CPSC's cancer risk assessment, though it was not necessary to decide them in order to vacate the CPSC action. Among these was the "questionable validity" of assuming the effective dose for humans is the same as for rats when exposure levels are the same. As discussed above, the issues of comparative metabolism and pharmacokinetics raises questions regarding limitations of current mathematical models as a basis for risk assessment.

It is apparent from the *Formaldehyde* case that the regulator needs as complete and objective a scientific evaluation as is possible in the circumstances. Many aspects of the assessment will involve judgments and uncertainties in gray areas. While the regulator may prefer black or white scientific findings, the partnership of law and science must be built on the kind of data and evaluations that are available within the current state of the art.

Simplistic use of mathematical models is not a satisfactory basis for regulatory decisions.

C. The Law is Not Concerned With Insignificant Risks

Life is not risk free. The principle that the law is not concerned with insignificant risks is embodied in the common law maxim *"de minimis non curat lex"*—the law is not concerned with trivialities. While Congress has the last word in the statutory arena and may indeed regulate or bar a trivial risk, courts have adopted principles of statutory interpretation based on the concept that the law deals with significant risks. That underlying principle of construction was stated recently in the *Benzene* case [1] holding that the Occupational Safety and Health Act applies only to "significant" risks.

Similarly, the U.S. Court of Appeals for the District of Columbia Circuit held that in applying the Delaney Clause's "unequivocal" ban on food additives that are shown by appropriate tests to induce cancer in animals, the FDA was not required to bar food containers from which small or *de minimis* amounts of a carcinogenic substance (in this acrylonitrile monomer) may migrate to the food [2].

The law faces the need for a means to determine which of the myriad and growing list of potential cancer risks are significant and which are trivial. The objective of a satisfactory working partnership must be a framework in which science can operate to inform the person or agency responsible for decision making so as to permit informed risk management judgments to identify and deal with significant risks. In the regulatory area, the partnership between law and science has developed most fully, often with the aid of the courts. We shall discuss next this developing partnership.

III. THE ROLE OF SCIENCE IN STATUTORY CONTROL OF CARCINOGENS

A. Statutory Developments

Statutes that have been adopted to control potential carcinogens have sometimes been divided into three general categories, based in part at least on the way science is used in the regulatory process [22] ; thus:

(i) Legislation that bans a *risk* when it is identified, *e.g.*, the Delaney Clause; (ii) legislation that *controls risks* by requiring use of a particular technology, *e.g.*, best practical or best available technology under the Clean Water Act; and (iii) legislation which *balances risk* against costs or benefits, *e.g.*, the Toxic Substances Control Act, which provides for regulation of unreasonable risks under a cost/benefit formula.

This categorization is useful, but in the present context it is perhaps more meaningful to consider how the statutory control options have changed as the need to develop a partnership of law and science has become clearer.

The first statute explicitly addressed to the risk of cancer was the Delaney Clause, adopted in 1958. Prior to that time, the Food and Drug Act, adopted in 1906, modernized by the Food, Drug and Cosmetic Act in 1938, generally provided that food may not contain "poisonous or deleterious substances which render it injurious to health."

In 1958, Congress adopted specific provisions dealing with food additives. Food additives are regulated under the general safety clause: the additive must be found safe under conditions of use specified in the regulation (21 U.S.C. § 348(c)(3)(A)). The 1958 amendment contained the Delaney Clause that provides that any food additive found to induce cancer in man or animals in an appropriate test may not be deemed safe (21 U.S.C. § 348(c)(3)(A)). In 1960, the Delaney Clause was extended to color additives (21 U.S.C. §§ 321(t) and 376(b)(5)(B)).

Finally, in the drug amendments of 1962 and the animal drug amendments of 1968, Congress adopted the so-called DES (diethylstilbestrol) proviso to the Delaney Clause with respect to residues of animal drugs in meat and meat products (21 U.S.C. § 360b(d)(1)(H)). Under the DES proviso, a carcinogenic animal drug can be used provided that a residue is not detected in the food products by an analytical method approved by the Commissioner of the FDA.

It should be emphasized that except for the specific prohibitions of the Delaney Clause, food safety decisions depend upon the exercise of good scientific judgment. Congress has not prohibited carcinogenic contaminants or constitutents (as opposed to intentional additives) in food. Control over contaminants or constituents is governed by the general safety provisions of the law, not the Delaney Clause.

The interaction of law and science in the regulation of food and drugs was modified by the anticancer prohibition of the Delaney Clause. While the Delaney Clause was ringed by exceptions, its concept was simple. If a food additive can be identified as cancer causing under the Delaney criteria, the size of the risk is unimportant (except for the *de mimimis* rule) and the substance must be banned.

The next stage in the interaction of law and science came with the adoption of the Clean Air Act in 1970 (42 U.S.C.A. § 7401 *et seq.*) and the Clean Water Act in 1972 (33 U.S.C. § 1251 *et seq.*). In those statutes, the risks to human health are, in general, controlled by specified levels of technology. While the technology requirements vary depending on the characterization of the risk, there is no gradation of control according to magnitude of risk except in general terms. For example, Section 301 of the Clean Water Act mandated effluent limitations by mandating the application of "best practical control technology currently available" by 1977 and "best available technology economically achievable" by 1983 (33 U.S.C. §§ 1311(b)(1)(A) and (2)(A)). The selection of the "best" technology implies some balancing of cost and benefit, but no adjustment for magnitude of risk.

The next stage in the evolution of the congressional approach involved the injection of a balancing of risks and benefits. In 1972, Congress adopted amendments to the Federal Insecticide, Fungicide and Rodenticide Act (FIFRA) which provided for control of pesticides based on a consideration of the benefits and risks of their uses (7 U.S.C. § 135 *et seq.*) Science played a role in the statutory plan for evaluating data relevant to both sides of that equation. The Clean Air Act Amendments of 1977 injected an element of balancing of risks against costs and feasibility in certain regulation of air omissions. However, § 112, which regulates hazardous air pollutants (including potential carcinogens), provides for control of toxic pollutants on the basis of health risks with an "ample margin of safety." Congress, however, did provide in § 117 for independent scientific review of the data and evaluations for regulatory decisions under § 112.

Finally, the Toxic Substances Control Act (TSCA), which became effective in 1977, deals specifically with carcinogens and establishes a procedure for balancing risks and benefits (15 U.S.C. § 2601 *et seq.*). The regulatory objective of TSCA is control of "unreasonable" risks.

The contrast between the zero risk provision of the Delaney clause and the balancing provisions of TSCA illustrate the growing understanding in the congress that science has a crucial role to play in the regulatory context by providing an assessment of the size and character of the risk, particularly where the issue is control of chronic health hazards such as carcinogens. The formation of the partnership of law and science has evolved to reflect the interaction contemplated between the scientist who evaluates the data and the regulator who must make the critical social/legal decisions.

B. The Legal Framework for Science: Peer Review and Independent Science Panels

While scientists sometimes participate in adversary proceedings in a court or before an administrative body, the method of scientific evaluation is normally nonadversarial. The objective of a scientific inquiry is usually described as consensus. Peer discussion and peer review are the devices used to test the relevance of data or the validity of an evaluation.

Congress has recognized this characteristic of the process of scientific evaluation. In the 1970 Clean Water Act, Congress provided for an independent scientific panel to review the adequacy of data for regulation of effluents under § 304 and new source standards under § 306. The Effluent Standard and Water Quality Information Advisory Committee created by § 515 was composed of a chairman and eight members selected on the basis of scientific training and experience. Appointed for a term of four years, the Committee held public meetings to receive comments on the data and evaluations to be used by the administrator. The Committee was not reappointed when the initial term expired.

Congress also perceived the need for independent peer review by science panels in other statutes. Science advisory committees were created under the Toxic Substances Control Act (15 U.S.C. § 2603(e)), the Clean Air Act (41 U.S.C.A. §§ 7409(d) and 7417), FIFRA (7 U.S.C. § 136w(d)), the Safe Drinking Water Act (42 U.S.C. § 300j-5), and the color additive provisions of the Delaney Clause (21 U.S.C. § 376). The EPA Science Advisory Board, of more general jurisdiction, originally created by administrative action, was given a statutory base by the Environmental Research, Development and Demonstration Authorization Act of 1978 (42 U.S.C. § 4365).

When the Consumer Products Safety Act was reauthorized in 1981, a Chronic Hazards Advisory Panel was created which must be consulted in regulatory actions involving risk of cancer, birth defects, or gene mutation (15 U.S.C. §§ 2077, 2080(b)).

In addition to these science advisory panels which were created by Congress as part of the regulatory pattern and which help to build the partnership of science, policy, and the law, many other agencies have advisory committees. None of these other committees has a continuing function of reviewing the adequacy of the science base for evaluating potential cancer risks, however.

C. The Report of the National Academy of Sciences (NAS) and the Recommendation of the Administrative Conference

In 1980 (P.L. 96-528), Congress appropriated funds to the Food and Drug Administration for a study of "alternative programs and institutional means to insure that federal regulatory policies with respect to carcinogens and other public health hazards of particular significance are developed on the basis of reliable scientific assessments" [23]. The results of the study [12] are a major contribution to both the methodology and the institutional means for conducting scientific risk assessments. Earlier in this chapter, some of the principle findings of the report were discussed.

The NAS study included a survey of the use of, and experience with, independent science panels by regulatory agencies and strongly recommended peer review by science panels as the best institutional means of assuring "reliable scientific assessment." Key recommendations of particular interest here include: preparation of a written risk assessment providing a review of scientific data (including health and exposure data) before any regulatory decision to regulate or not to regulate, and review of the agency risk assessments by an independent science advisory panel before any major regulatory action or decision not to regulate.

The NAS report concluded that where peer review by an independent science panel is mandated, the agencies "produce final risk assessments in support of regulatory decisions that are generally of high scientific quality and are accepted by the public and the regulated parties." The report recommended that where independent science panels already exist, they should be used to review scientific risk evaluations. Where none exist, the report recommends that panels be created.

Pursuant to the basic concept of separation between scientific risk assessment and the function of risk management, the report proposes that scientific or technical competence be the basis for choice of members of a panel; it recommends against organizational affiliation as a basis for selection.

To emphasize the distinction between risk assessment and risk management, the report concludes that "[i]f risk management considerations (for example, the economic or political effects of a particular control action for a particular chemical) are seen to affect . . . the scientific interpretations . . . in a risk assessment, the credibility of the assessment inside and outside the agency can be compromised, and the risk management decision itself may lose legitimacy."

The Administrative Conference of the United States (ACUS) has also recommended peer review of the scientific basis for regulatory decisions on carcinogens [24]. ACUS concluded:

Peer review of experimental findings and scientific judgments is an important means of validating the technical bases of regulatory decisions concerning carcinogens.

ACUS also recommended that to the extent compatible with law, agencies should structure their decision processes to incorporate mechanisms for scientific peer review, noting that

> Advisory panels can contribute objectivity as well as expertise to agency decisions. Their advice has sometimes prevented erroneous regulatory actions; more frequently, their role has been to illuminate complex issues and enhance the quality, and thus the credibility, of agency scientific analysis.

Clearly, incorporating the recommendations of the NAS and the ACUS into the regulatory process will improve the developing partnership which is the subject of this chapter.

D. Pending Proposed Legislation

Over the years there have been proposals to create a central science panel that would complement or supplant the agency independent science panels discussed above. The NAS Report provided a new focus for legislative initiative. Building on the NAS Report a new bill, H.R. 4192, has been introduced as of this writing (December 1983) in the 98th Congress to establish a central science panel. The proposal recognizes the important role of agency science panels in assuring the adequacy of the regulatory science base and provides review by a central science panel only of those risk assessments made by agencies that involve scientific issues of national importance. The determination of importance would be by the involved agency and would require the concurrence of the Directors of the Office of Science and Technology Policy (OSTP) and the National Academy of Sciences (NAS).

H.R. 4192 builds on the framework that Congress has provided for the interaction of science and the law. The proposals would further implement two basic propositions: first, society cannot intelligently regulate substances that present human risks and benefits without having an estimate of the magnitude and character of the risk; and second, nonadversarial, objective science, including use of the scientific process of peer review, is the means which has evolved for incorporating good science into the regulatory process.

E. The Regulatory Experience

Developments in the interaction of the law and science in the regulatory arena have occurred mostly within the last six or seven years; the partnership between law and science in the agencies is still in the process of evolution. While the history of development is not smooth, the results have been good, and the outlook for the future is favorable.

1. Occupational Safety and Health Administration

Section 6(b) of the OSH Act directs the Secretary to set a standard for toxic materials "which most adequately assures, to the extent feasible, on the basis of the best available evidence, that no employee will suffer material impairment of health or functional capacity...." (29 U.S.C. § 655(b)(5)). Section 3(8), (29 U.S.C. § 652(8)), provides that the standards under the Act shall be based on "the latest available scientific data in the field...."

The NAS Report made the following evaluation of OSHA's risk evaluation procedures: "OSHA historically has done a less thorough job than other agencies in obtaining relevant scientific information and independent peer review of this information before issuing a notice of proposed rule-making... OSHA's use of rule-making proceedings to provide scientific review stands in sharp contrast with the other agencies' procedures for review. In the [NAS] Committee's opinion, this reliance on public proceedings to strengthen and refine the scientific basis for the agency's regulatory actions has not been an adequate substitute for independent peer review."

On October 4, 1977, OSHA published a draft of a proposed generic cancer regulation (42 *Fed. Reg.* 54148). There were extensive hearings in 1978, and on January 22, 1980, a final generic regulation was published. (45 *Fed. Reg.* 5002).

The OSHA generic regulation provided a formal scheme for identifying and classifying potential occupational carcinogens. By administrative fiat, OSHA directed what regulatory significance should be attributed to certain classes of experimental data, particularly positive animal studies. The regulation forced the scientific evaluations into a yes/no category. If the data on a substance satisfied the inflexible regulatory criteria, the substance was to be regulated as a carcinogen. No quantification of risk was attempted (except for prioritization), and the level of regulation was fixed at the lowest feasible limit or at zero if substitutes were available. Regulatory decisions were required without distinction between trivial and significant risks.

The NAS Report made the following comment on the generic rule:

> The final rule did not address exposure assessment and rejected the use of dose-response assessment for any regulatory purpose except priority-setting. . . . For reasons of efficiency, the guidelines were written in language that permitted little deviation from the judgments embodied in them.

Shortly after the generic regulation was published, the Supreme Court set aside the OSHA benzene standard which followed the precepts of the generic regulation [1]. As indicated earlier, the Court held that OSHA may not adopt a standard under § 6(b) until it has made a threshold finding that there is a significant risk—for benzene, a significant risk of cancer—at the levels of exposure found in the workplace. Moreover, the Court concluded that OSHA could not adopt a standard without a finding that the standard will significantly reduce the risk.

In the subsequent *Cotton Dust* decision [25], the Court held that a *general* risk/benefit analysis is not required under the OSH Act. However, the Court reaffirmed the ruling in *Benzene* that OSHA must find both that a significant risk exists at workplace exposure levels and that a significant reduction can be achieved under the feasibility criteria of the law before regulation of carcinogens is authorized under the OSH Act.

Following the *Benzene* decision, OSHA began a reconsideration of the generic regulation. Critical parts of the regulation inconsistent with *Benzene* were deleted on January 19, 1981 (46 *Fed. Reg.* 4889). On January 5, 1982, OSHA published an Advance Notice of Proposed Rule Making (ANPR) for review of the generic regulation (47 *Fed. Reg.* 187). The reconsideration is not complete as of this writing (December, 1983).

2. Environmental Protection Agency

EPA has done more than other agencies to establish systematic procedures for independent scientific review of the adequacy of the data base for regulation of potential carcinogens. Review of the scientific base of regulatory action by the Science Advisory Panel is mandated by § 25(d) of FIFRA (7 U.S.C. § 136w(e)). The Clean Air Act mandated review by the independent scientific committee established under § 117 of the scientific basis for regulatory decisions under §§ 108, 111, 112, and 202. The agency-wide EPA Science Advisory Board (SAB), originally established by administrative order, now has a statutory base. However, in contrast to review by the Science Advisory Panel under FIFRA, review by the SAB of the science base for agency action is a matter determined by the Administrator. The same is true of the use of science panels under § 109(d)(2) of the Clean Air Act.

In addition to independent science advisory committees created under the statutes EPA administers, the EPA administrator issued two orders providing for independent peer review of the validity of the science base. Order #2200, dated October 9, 1981, provided for peer review of documents, data, reports, publications, and contracts [26]. And in February 1982, the administrator issued a guideline memorandum which established a new set of requirements for scientific review by the Science Advisory Board of significant EPA regulatory actions [27].

The partnership interactions of the scientific risk assessment function and the legal/regulatory functions continue to develop. In the meantime, EPA has taken important steps to ensure the adequacy of the science base for its regulatory decisions.

3. Food and Drug Administration

FDA has many independent science panels, though only in one instance is review by a science panel dealing with potential carcinogens legislatively mandated. The Delaney clause provisions of the color additive provisions of the food safety laws provide for the appointment of an ad hoc scientific advisory committee, selected by the National Academy of Sciences, upon request by a person adversely affected by an order on color additives (21 U.S.C. 376(b)(5)(D)). There does not appear to be any significant experience under this provision.

Nitrites, mentioned earlier, present an example of an ad hoc FDA science panel to review the experimental basis for proposed regulation of a potential carcinogen. Nitrites are important for the control of botulism bacteria in meats. In August of 1978, FDA received a report of an animal study on the potential carcinogenicity of nitrites. The study was reported to be positive, allegedly showing an increase in lymphoma in rats fed nitrites in their diet. FDA and the Department of Agriculture announced plans to phase out the use of nitrites prior to peer review of the study. Two years later, after a thorough peer review, the study was found to be negative rather than positive as originally reported. In the two years required to evaluate the study, both a significant amount of publicity and public controversy and a considerable expenditure of funds by industry and government occurred. The history of the nitrites case was a factor in the decision by the Congress to appropriate funds for a study which finally led to the preparation of the NAS report.

4. Interagency Cooperation

In 1977, the four regulatory agencies (EPA, FDA, OSHA, and CPSC, later joined by the Department of Agriculture) formed the Interagency Regulatory Liaison Group (IRLG). One of the important products of that effort was the publication of a draft scientific report on cancer in July 1979 (44 *Fed. Reg.* 39858). The report was never peer reviewed by independent scientists. Extensive public comments were received, but the comments were never reviewed by the IRLG nor was the draft revised as had been promised.

A new effort at interagency cooperation is now under way under the auspices of the President's Office of Science and Technology Policy. Scientists from the regulatory agencies, together with their counterparts from the National Center for Toxicological Research and the National Institute for Environmental Health Sciences, are preparing two scientific documents on cancer: a "state-of-the-art" document on cancer and a "principles" document for use by the agencies. The success and acceptability of this effort will turn on the effective use of scientific peer review and a full opportunity for public comment.

IV. NEW OPPORTUNITIES FOR THE PARTNERSHIP OF LAW AND SCIENCE

There has been much criticism that both the law and the regulatory process are slow, cumbersome, and costly. This has been the case particularly when addressing chronic health hazards such as cancer. An opportunity to deal with this criticism by extending the partnership of law and science arises from the move to substitute a negotiated approach in the regulatory arena for the present confrontational procedure. Some progress has already been made.

The adoption of the Administrative Procedure Act in 1946 (5 U.S.C. § 551 *et seq.*) marked a major advance in dealing with federal rule making. The distinction between adjudicative proceedings, which take on the character of judicial litigation, and the legislative, informal rule-making process was an important step forward. Both procedures, however, included the confrontational mode of dealing with scientific issues. While confrontation has been tempered where an independent science panel acts successfully, the mode of confrontation remains a characteristic of the regulatory process.

Milton Wessel has written extensively on the problems and opportunities of developing a consensus by negotiation [28]. Wessel takes the position that credible "good science" is what is needed for the resolution of what he calls "socio-scientific disputes" that involve quality-of-life issues. Unfortunately, the normal development of a scientific consensus, which is essentially voluntary, takes an undue amount of time. Wessel therefore proposes that a state-of-the-science conference be convened in the regulatory process to provide a sound science base for negotiated dispute resolution.

More novel yet, the Administrative Conference of the United States (ACUS) and, on an experimental basis, EPA and OSHA have considered the viability of a procedure for negotiation among representatives of the parties interested in a regulation. This goes well beyond the scientific area, penetrating to social areas of risk management and control. The most complete formal proposal of negotiated regulation was prepared and presented for comment by ACUS and subsequently published as a final recommendation in July 1982 [29]. The recommendation deals with the details of negotiation: identification of the parties and the issues ripe for negotiation, conduct of negotiation, selection of agency representative as convenor, etc.

These proposals for consensus science and, more far-reaching yet, regulatory negotiation (based on consensus science) in the regulatory process are still in the opportunity stage. The possibilities for success in integrating risk assessment and peer review into the regulatory process raises hope and expectations that the partnership will be expanded into this new arena. If regulatory negotiations can be successful—and the concept is fraught with perceived obstacles at this time—the entire regulatory process may be improved and concerns for its cumbersomeness and cost allayed. Only earnest future efforts can aim this new departure toward success.

V. CONCLUSION

As pointed out at the outset of this chapter, there is a fundamental similarity between the concept of causality in law and science. Both deal with fact and with gradations based on probability. There are differences in the institutional settings in which the concepts apply; however, close analysis shows the similarities.

In the legal system there are degrees of proof: preponderance of the evidence, or proof beyond a reasonable doubt. The law is also concerned with whether the cause is proximate or remote. All of these concepts are designed to sort out the gradations of fact and cause based on concepts similar to the concepts of probability common in scientific evaluations.

Both law and science must make sharp distinctions. In law, the decision must be made as to causality. In science, the evaluation which may be in general terms becomes specific when the doctor or clinician makes a diagnosis. In both law and science, the more that is known about the mechanism of the disease or injury, the greater the assurance of the correctness of the decision. Neither demands absolute proof; the institution and the procedure may be different, but the basic concepts of causation and the need for making decisions in the midst of "uncertainty" are similar.

There is an obvious need for a mechanism to ensure that objective scientific consensus is available to courts and juries in the rising tide of environmental and product litigation. Congress and the states are considering legislative proposals to by-pass the traditional legal processes. There is a possible basis of a partnership of law and science that provides an alternative to radical legislative proposals. Such a partnership could be based on the concept in the Federal Rules of Evidence of court-appointed expert witnesses on scientific issues [30]. A mechanism for identification and compensation for such objective scientific witnesses needs to be worked out.

Important beginnings have been made in creating new legal frameworks in which consensus science can make important contributions to the resolution of regulatory issues. The credibility of regulatory decisions that are perceived to be based on sound, unbiased science suggests that there will be an extension of nonconfrontational methods for resolving scientific regulatory issues. The success in the regulatory area offers hope that a procedure such as court-appointed expert witnesses will emerge for presenting scientific consensus that does not require a radical change in the long legal tradition that has handled private disputes with reasonable success and dispatch.

Developments to date have not been smooth. They have none-theless moved in the direction of improving the relationship of science and the law in the areas in which they can mutually assist each other in reducing the risks of industrially derived cancer. There is every reason to hope for further, constructive develop-ment of the partnership between science, policy, and the law in the future and, therefore, for continuing success in reducing in-dustrially related cancer risk.

REFERENCES

1. *Industrial Union Department* v. *American Petroleum Institute*, 448 U.S. 607 (1980).
2. *Monsanto Co.* v. *Kennedy*, 613 F. 2d 947 (D.C. Cir. 1979).
3. David P. Rall, quoted in an article entitled "Toxic-waste fights start in laboratories, but how good are the testing methods" *The Wall Street Journal*, June 21, 1983.
4. Lewis Thomas, *Youngest Science*, The Viking Press, 1983. [Published as part of the Alfred P. Sloan Foundation Science Program.]
5. Elizabeth K. Weisburger, History of the bioassay program of the Nation-al Cancer Institute, *Prog. Exp. Tumor Res., 26*:187-201 (1983).
6. National Institute of Occupational Safety and Health, U.S.D.H.E.W. *Suspected Carcinogens: A Subfile of the NIOSH Toxic Substances List* (1976).
7. *Federal Register, 48*:35508 (August 4, 1983).
8. David P. Rall, Statement Before the Subcommittee on Departmental Operations, Research and Foreign Agriculture of the House Committee on Agriculture, July 27, 1983.
9. R. D. Bruce, *et al.*, Reexamination of the ED_{01} Study: Audit of Pathol-ogy, *Fund, and Appl. Toxicol., 1*:27-128 (1981). [See also Philippe Shubik, Objective of Carcinogenicity Testing, *Fund. and Appl. Toxicol., 3*:137 (1983).]
10. *Federal Register, 47*:52140 (November 19, 1982).
11. *Federal Register, 47*:53843 (November 30, 1983); *Federal Register 48*: 5252 (February 4, 1983).
12. National Research Council, *Risk Assessment in the Federal Government: Managing the Process*, Committee on the Institutional Means for Assess-ment of Risks to Public Health, National Academy Press, Washington, D.C. (1983).

13. William D. Ruckelshaus, Science, risk and public policy, address to the National Academy of Sciences, June 22, 1983, reprinted in the *Daily Congressional Record*, Vol. 129, p. S9356 (June 28, 1983).
14. Office of Science and Technology Policy, Executive Office of the President, *Identification, Characterization and Control of Potential Carcinogens: A Framework for Federal Decision Making*, February 1, 1979. [Reprinted in the *J. Nat'l Cancer Inst., 61*:169-175 (January 1980).]
15. *Federal Register, 46*:15501 (March 6, 1981).
16. David G. Hoel, Norman L. Kaplan, Marshall W. Anderson, Implications of non-linear kinetics on risk estimation in carcinogenesis, *Science, 219*: 1032-1037 (March 1983).
17. Testimony of Kenneth S. Crump, Ph.D., OSHA hearings on ethylene oxide, prepared statement at 26 (July 1983) OSHA Docket No. H-200.
18. Robert A. Squire, *Science, 219*:236-238 (January 21, 1983).
19. *A Report on the Workshop on Biological and Statistical Implications of the ED$_{01}$ Study and Related Data Bases*, workshop sponsored by the National Center for Toxicological Research and the Society of Toxicology, September 13-16, 1981, Deer Creek State Park, Mt. Sterling, Ohio. *Fund. and Appl. Toxicol., 3*:129-160 (1983).
20. Robert A. Squire, Ranking animal carcinogens: A proposed regulatory approach, *Science, 214*:877-880 (November 20, 1981).
21. *Gulf South Insulation* v. *United States Consumer Product Safety Commission*, 701 F. 2d 1137 (5th Cir. 1983), *rehearing denied, id.*
22. Office of Technology Assessment, *Assessment of Technologies for Determining Cancer Risks from the Environment* (June 1981). [See esp. Chapt. VI, "Approaches to Regulating Carcinogens," pp. 175-208.]
23. S. Rep. No. 96-1030, 96th Cong., 2nd Sess. (p. 99).
24. Administrative Conference of the United States, Recommendation 82-5, *Federal Regulation of Cancer-Causing Chemicals, Fed. Reg. 47*:30701 (July 15, 1982).
25. *American Textile Manufacturers Institute* v. *Donovan*, 452 U.S. 490 (1981).
26. Environmental Protection Agency (EPA), *Peer Review Process for Scientific and Informational Documents* (October 9, 1981).
27. Environmental Protection Agency, Memorandum to Assistant Administrators, Associate Administrators and Office Directors on "Improving the Scientific Adequacy of Agency Regulations and Standards", February 1982.
28. Milton R. Wessel, The "State of the Science" Conference: A New Approach to Scientific Decision Making, *Fund. Appl. Toxicol. 2*:283-288 (1982).

29. U.S. Administrative Conference, *Proposed Recommendation Procedure for Negotiating Proposed Regulations*, request for public comments, *Fed. Reg.*, 47:11024, (March 15, 1982); Recommendation 82-4, 1 CFR § 305.82-4, *Fed. Reg.*, 47:30701, 30708 (July 15, 1982). See Also: Philip J. Harter, "Negotiating Regulations: A Cure for the Malaise?" (1982) available from the Office of the Chairman, Administrative Conference of the United States, 2120 L Street, NW, Washington, D.C. 20037.

30. Federal Rules of Evidence § 706. The Advisory Committee characterized the inherent power of a trial judge to call his own experts as "virtually unquestioned." Notes of Advisory Committee on Proposed Rules, Comment on Federal Rule of Evidence 706. See also "The Present Status of the Impartial Medical Experts in Civil Litigation," 34 Temple L.Q476 (1961); and David W. Peck, "Impartial Medical Testimony," 22 F.R.O.21 (1959).

INDEX